GET THE F*CK UNSTUCK!

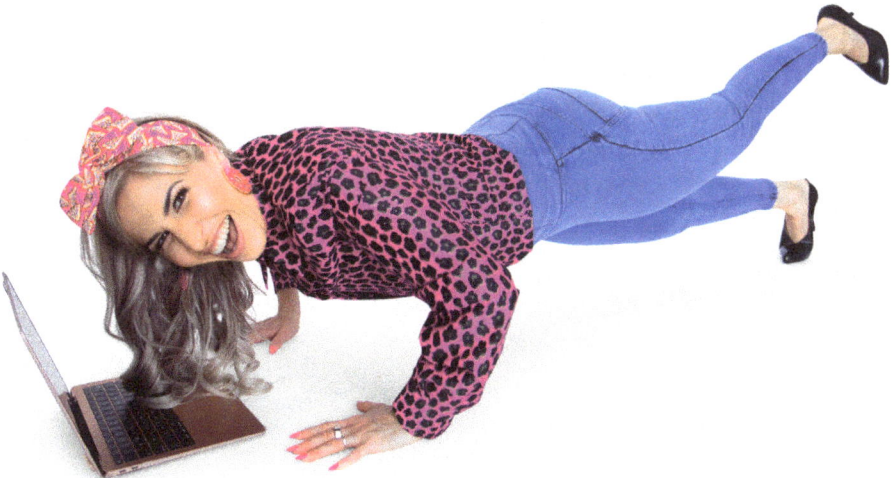

Throughout, Antonenko offers a supportive voice that enthusiastically urges the reader to "design the life of your dreams." The advice is largely a mix of generic tips for healthy living (such as getting enough sleep, embracing mindfulness, eating a balanced diet, including minimizing consumption of sugars and processed food) and common self-help bromides about visualizing success and ignoring what other people think. However, Antonenko wisely focuses on permanently changing behaviors rather than promoting expedient solutions that may be harder to stick with in the long term. The book includes links to supplemental material on the author's website, such as printable affirmation cards, a meal planner, and a separate exercise guide. This work stands well enough on its own, but it's also intended as an introduction to Antonenko's life-coaching offerings, which include follow-up courses, fitness accessories, and nutritional supplements.

An earnest and straightforward, if familiar, guide to transforming one's routines.

– Kirkus Indie Reviews, Austin, Texas.

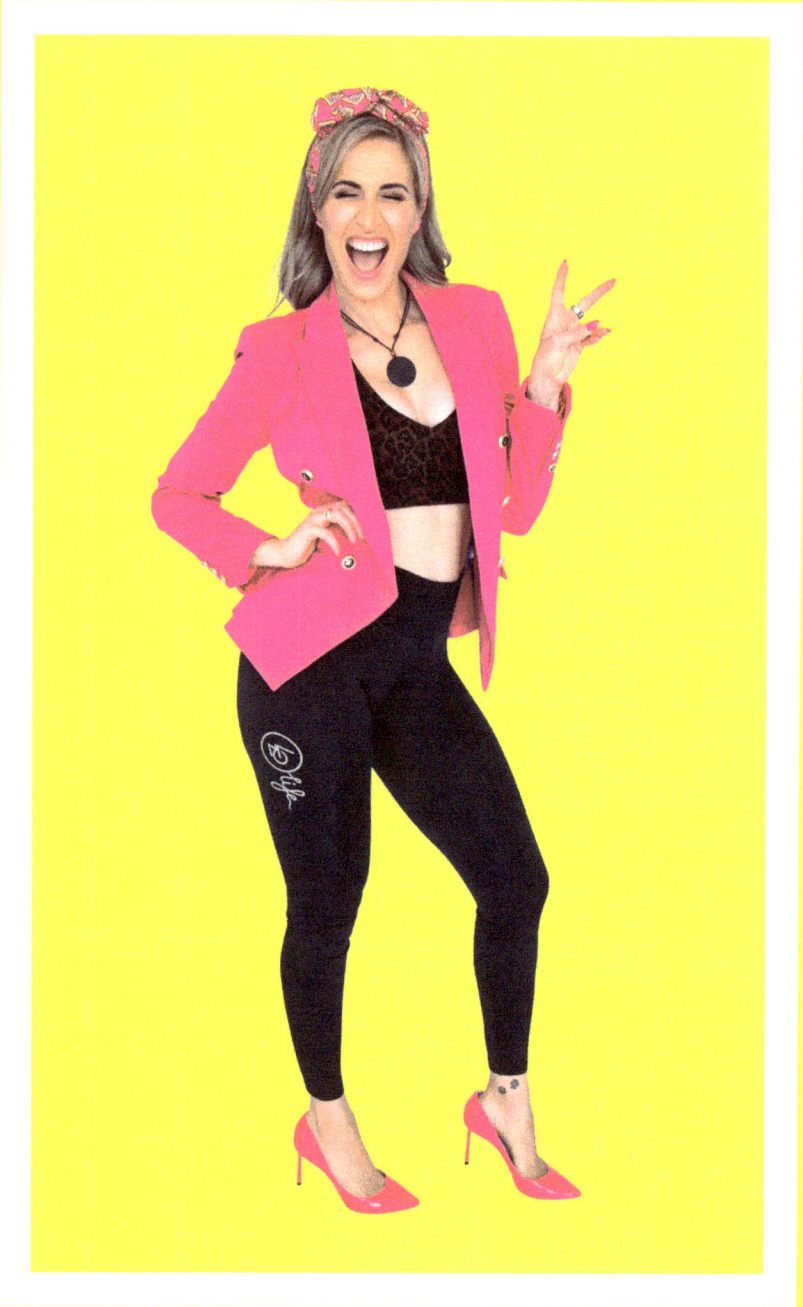

GET THE F*CK UNSTUCK!

A BS-Free Healthy Habit Handbook for Busy People to Take Their Lives from Stuck to Unstoppable

Loz Antonenko

First published in 2024 by Dean Publishing
PO Box 119
Mt. Macedon, Victoria, 3441
Australia
deanpublishing.com

DEAN PUBLISHING

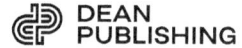

Cataloguing-in-Publication Data
National Library of Australia
Title: Get The F*ck Unstuck! A BS-Free Healthy Habit Handbook for Busy People to Take Their Lives from Stuck to Unstoppable
Edition: 1st edn
ISBN: 978-1-925452-85-3
Category: Health/Fitness/Nutrition

Diagrams and "Loz Lesson" images have
been designed using images from Flaticon.com

CONTENTS

Introduction 1

Quick Start Guide 15

It's Okay to Feel Stuck 19

The Basics 43

Momentum 59

Menu 99

Mindset 131

Movement 175

Mastery 195

Mentorship 209

Closing Words 232

IRL (In Real Loz) 235

Acknowledgements 240

About the Author 244

Endnotes 247

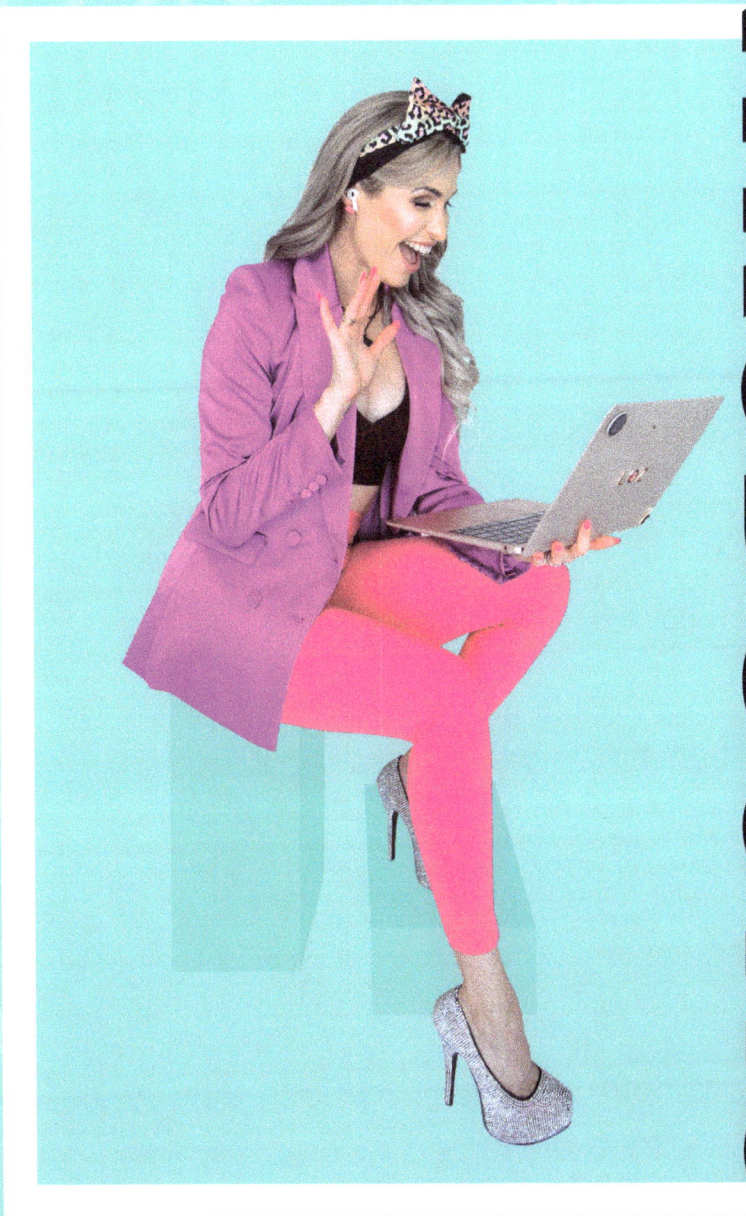

INTRODUCTION

WANNA GET THE F*CK UNSTUCK?

Hands up if you have tried a diet, attempted meditation, or flogged yourself silly with exercise but never got the results you expected or wanted. Perhaps you, with good intentions, bought all the fabulous activewear and signed up for a gym membership you didn't use.

If that *is* you, don't be hard on yourself. You're not alone.

Having been there myself, I know what it feels like to lack motivation. I understand what it's like to crave change and not know how to achieve the lifestyle and health outcomes I dream of.

But achieving those goals is possible – I promise!

Ask yourself these questions.

* Am I so busy trying to juggle work, family, relationships, and health that I have become stuck?

* Do I need help deciphering and putting all available health and diet information into a cohesive and actionable plan?

* Am I ready to take action to get myself unstuck?

If you answered yes, yes, yes, this handbook of healthy habits is the perfect tool to guide you through the hurdles and through a blueprint to live your life to the fullest. You've just entered a BS-free zone. In *Get the F*ck Unstuck!,* you will learn practical and simple ways to cultivate loving kindness, find meaningful motivation, and commit to creating positive, lifelong habits.

Before we get down to business, I want to share a bit about myself. My journey has been far from smooth. In fact, it has been about as rough as they come. If you're feeling lost or hopeless right now, I want you to know I've been there before in a *big* way, but, through building healthy habits, I managed to get the f*ck unstuck – and you can too.

MY STORY

As a child, I always knew I would live an extraordinary life. I vividly recall repeatedly telling my parents that I would achieve something incredible throughout this lifetime. My life purpose fluctuated between becoming a famous actor, discovering some distant galaxy, and finding the key to a scientific breakthrough. Either way, my hyperactive imagination connected me to the profound feeling that my life would involve something significant.

If you told the 21-year-old me that I would be where I am today, living a far-from-average life, and described to me the immense heartaches and triumphs that would take place along the way, there is no chance that I would have taken you seriously. It has been one hell of a journey, but here I am as walking, talking proof that you can move from stuck to unstoppable!

In 2010, believe it or not, my life was very average. I ran a family business with my father, and I was about to get married to the most caring, loving, giving person I had ever met – Brian.

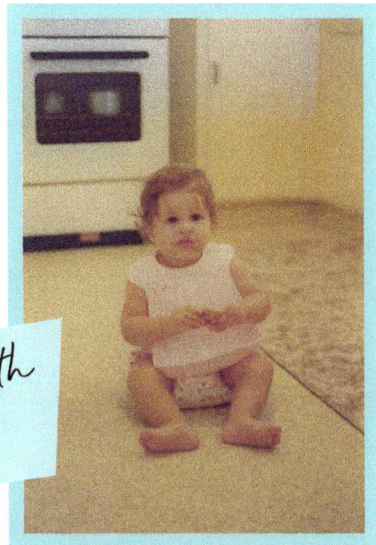

I swear I was born with food in my mouth!

Together, we lived under the roof of my family home and saved a significant deposit to build our first home because we didn't want to rent. My father had always taught me the importance of money and how much it dictated your quality of life (but more about this later). Dad educated me about investing for my future and encouraged me to read books like Robert Kiyosaki's *Rich Dad Poor Dad* while I was an impressionable teenager. I'm grateful for that.

As young adults, Brian and I owned every tangible object that we thought would provide us with happiness. From the outside, I seemed to have my shit together, and, subsequently, I lived a very predictable, secure, and confident life.

My husband-to-be and I shared a deep connection. We had been living together with my family for five years, sacrificing our personal space and privacy to save money so we could get ahead. While I worked in the family business, my fiancé worked for a government department.

Our shared love of adventure meant we spent our weekends kayaking, four-wheel driving, and going out on weekly dinner dates – the kinds of things you do when life is good. We did everything together and depended on each other to fill our love buckets. And they were packed!

While Brian was focused on ascending the hierarchy at work and improving his body and mind at the gym, I was dedicated to learning the art of running a small business. I was very grateful to be recognised by the local business community with various awards. These accolades helped to externally validate my actions by providing me with an assured sense of significance – more on that need for external validation later.

At the same time, I was struggling with my health, having been diagnosed with ulcerative colitis. This debilitating autoimmune condition causes the body's immune system to create inflammation and ulcers in the bowel, with arthritic-like symptoms of pain throughout the body. When it flares up, life is absolutely physically and emotionally overwhelming. I also suffered from polycystic ovary syndrome, pyrrole disorder, premenstrual dysphoric disorder, a tumour on my pituitary gland, and depression, among many other labels given to me by medical professionals.

Luckily, what doesn't kill us makes us stronger, right? If only it were that easy.

Subsequently, my self-esteem was at an all-time low, and a long stint of steroidal medication caused me to gain much weight over a short period. What did this look like? Most of my weight gain was in my lower abdomen, buttocks, and the backs of my arms, so the labels 'barge arse' and 'dump truck' come to mind. To compensate for my bottom-heavy, oestrogen-dominant body shape, I dressed conservatively, wearing loose-fitting clothing to mask my ample backside and tiny, boobless chest.

Nonetheless, Brian loved me for me. No matter what, he told me daily that he loved me and empathised with me and the constant struggle I found in existing. He really was an incredible partner. Even so, our relationship wasn't perfect.

Stuck as F*ck

In my mind, we were a happy couple with a beautiful future ahead. However, Brian and I were both silently battling mental health challenges. Our relationship was super co-dependent, and we didn't autonomously develop any personal coping strategies to help us overcome tough times. I've always considered myself quite stubborn and stoic, but Brian? No, he was like a Caramello

Koala: hard on the outside but soft and gooey on the inside. Unfortunately, a tough, hardened external façade can mask what's happening inside.

After two rounds of plastic surgery – the first one in 2014 to fix a deviated septum and change my nose while they were at it, and the second in 2015 to 'grow' some boobs – my confidence hit a new high. Brian, though, was trying to manage frustration after frustration. He was struggling to find his sense of purpose, and, in his search, forfeited his stable, long-term employment within the government to pursue a more exciting job in the private sector. Then he lost his job. His confidence plummeted, and I was the only person to whom he divulged his pain and suffering. If only he had let others into his internal turmoil. I didn't know it at the time, but the real challenges were just beginning.

In late 2015, my father and I had a physical altercation at work. We had been in business together, running our family mobility equipment store, since 2007, and he was in the depths of an existential crisis. Amid a divorce from my mother after nearly three decades of marriage, his ability to cope was severely compromised. When a bedpan didn't have a price on it, I somehow copped the blame, and this seemingly insignificant incident escalated to a physical outburst of anger where I was struck in the face. I was scared, confused, and concerned for my family's safety. After months of blame and harassment, I was forced to completely disengage from his toxic behaviour. Although I had spent my entire life trying to prove myself to him to earn his love and respect and had forged a value system based on his high expectations of me, my father has not spoken to me since this time, and he has written me out of his will and scratched me from his history.

Just when I thought life couldn't get any more difficult…

Two days after my 31st birthday, Brian committed suicide. Instead of celebrating my birthday, I drove with my family and his mum to Boonah, where he had jumped off Mount French in front of his dad and sister. This is where I saw his lifeless body. Up to this point in my life, I hadn't even lost a close family member, and I never in a million years thought the first person I would lose would be the first great love of my life.

To top off this period of immense heartache, a short month later, my aged but significantly cognitive paternal grandfather passed away in hospital after a short battle with ill health. At his small funeral, I again faced my father, who didn't speak to me. But more challenges were to come.

As a consequence of this shitshow trifecta, as you can imagine, life became far more complicated – emotionally, mentally, and physically. Naturally, I struggled to come to terms with Brian's passing and the loss of my two paternal father figures. I was utterly heartbroken, confused, and overwhelmed with conflicting emotions. I lost my identity, my purpose, and my sense of belonging.

I was the definition of 'stuck'.

Moving from Stuck to Unstoppable

Fast forward to today, and my life has been turned on its head.

I've built a thriving, million-dollar family business, climbed the tallest freestanding mountain in the world, skydived over a glacier, become a successful social media influencer, and competed in bodybuilding competitions… just for fun.

To top it all off, in my 30s, I discovered – and had repaired – a hole in my heart.

Now married to Michael, I have inherited a stepdaughter and am grateful to be a grandmother by proxy (affectionately known as 'G-Ma'). How cool is all of that?

Since writing the first version of this book, I have started a new, exciting chapter of my life as a personal trainer, life coach, professional speaker, business coach, and wellness advocate.

I have committed to 'me-search' over 'research'.

My business, Loz Life, has provided me with a platform to help many people move from stuck to unstoppable by harnessing the transformative power of daily routine and habits. My mission is to help busy people upgrade their happiness, health, and vitality to take them from stuck to unstoppable.

With my team of energised coaches, Loz Life inspires purposeful, mission-driven people to prioritise their eating, breathing, sleep, movement, and hydration so they can live longer, happier, more fulfilled lives, with energy, focus, and confidence.

Although I still struggle with my health, I am the fittest, most fulfilled, and most fabulous I have ever been. Enduring adversity has imprinted stoicism in my character and helped me build resilience. It has also gifted me with perspective. I live with purpose and presence and have more clarity than ever before. I am the master of my mind, body, and life. Pretty sweet, huh?

As you can see, once upon a time, I was where you may be right now – thinking the same shitty thoughts, making the same toxic judgements, feeling the same repetitive frustrations, and getting in my own way.

In a nutshell, my tumultuous journey has been heartbreakingly life-changing in so many ways. Despite these challenges, I have simplified to amplify. I have released the handbrakes that held me back from unleashing my ability to add value to the lives of others through service above self by focusing on some really basic daily habits. I now know that I endured all of this heartbreak for one purpose: to help people like you and me move from stuck to unstoppable. To go from merely surviving to thriving!

Through loss and suffering, I have realised that the ultimate key to long-term resilience, fulfilment, joy, and success lies in the intricacies of establishing healthy, habit-forming practices in our daily lives. It's actually pretty simple once you start, but that's the part most people suck at – *starting*.

LET'S DO THIS

I bet you've picked up this book because you realised you are stuck somewhere in your life. It's not an *accident* that you have been drawn to me and my story at this time in your life.

Maybe you have hit a period of stagnation in your life journey, identified that you are 'over it', and stumbled across this book because you are looking for answers. Perhaps you were intrigued by the title (yes, I'm mad for an f-bomb, in case you missed it) on your quest to improve your vitality as you consider your mortality. Or maybe you feel like everyone around you is progressing forward and winning in their lives, and you're just stuck in the same patterns you've been repeating for the past however many years.

Too many of us are exhausted all the time. We feel lethargic, tired, overly busy, stretched to breaking, and stressed without any time to focus on feeling good. We're so busy giving ourselves to everyone around us – our family, our friends, our careers – that we're left with nothing in the tank. It feels like we're driving around with the hand-brake on, right?

Commit to your 'me-search'

Just getting through your day can feel like pushing a giant rock up a mountain, and let's be honest – we're over feeling like crap every day! But don't we all feel a little guilty, maybe even a tad selfish, for taking some time out for ourselves?

I call BS on that! The reality is: You. Are. Worth. It. And guess what? You already hold the solution in your hands.

By picking up this book, you've taken the first step towards creating a more sustainable and healthy life… *congratulations*! Reading the pages ahead will be an easy task, but what won't be easy is actioning change in your life.

Sorry, friends, there's no quick fix.

The challenge of action separates the go-getters from the 'round-to-its', and *that's* the difference between living an extraordinary life and a life of regretful inaction.

At this divinely timed moment, I welcome you to the incredible journey of the *rest of your life*. How cool is that?

No matter how challenging, I promise you it is *always* worth it. There is no higher achievement nor more fulfilling gift that you can give yourself – and the world – than mastering your mind, body, and life, moving from stuck to unstoppable, and living your best life. Take heed from all those friendly dogs you see with their heads hanging out car windows, letting the air rush past their faces as they live in the moment. That could be you!

From the depths of my soul, I am infinitely grateful for the wisdom I have acquired throughout my life, and I look forward to helping you learn how to gain control of your emotions. By expanding our energy to a higher place of love, compassion, and unwavering authenticity, we all possess the capacity to live an extraordinary life and inspire others to do the same.

ARE YOU READY?

I want you to know that I'm super excited and feel privileged that you've chosen to engage with my book. I'm on a mission to help you learn loving kindness, meaningful motivation, and heartfelt commitment to creating positive, lifelong habits. You, too, can absolutely move from feeling stuck to unstoppable.

I hope you'll help share this mission with others by reading and studying the chapters carefully and then going out and living your learnings daily through inspired action. And don't be hard on yourself if you trip and fall along the way. My Loz Life community is here to support you, and so am I!

To help you connect and stay inspired, I'd love to invite you to follow my journey on social media.

* Facebook page: www.facebook.com/LozAntonenko

* LinkedIn profile: www.linkedin.com/in/lozantonenko/

* Instagram: www.instagram.com/lozantonenko

I cannot wait to share with you all the best advice I have gathered through my extensive experience. The time for wishing and waiting is over because right now, in this perfect moment, it is your time to take action.

Right, then – it's time to get the f*ck unstuck!

Loz Lesson

Do you know how I talked about doing the work? Well, it starts within the pages of this book. Throughout each chapter, I've included some healthy habits homework, each titled 'Loz Lesson', with links to printables, posters, and other super helpful tools.

Before we dive right into it, please download and print the **Positive Affirmation Cards** and put them around your house and/or workplace. Let these small reminders help you affirm your self-worth and dedication towards this meaningful self-development journey that you are about to embark on.

Words are so powerful! Some of my affirmations are:

☆ I accept myself exactly as I am now.

☆ I am valuable.

☆ I appreciate everything I have.

☆ I trust in my body's power to heal.

☆ If I can imagine it, I can achieve it.

☆ I am thankful for all the love in my life.

☆ I can forgive.

☆ I am safe.

Seriously, you should be super proud of taking this step. It's a big one. I've got you!

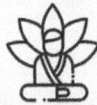

LOZ'S POSITIVE AFFIRMATION CARDS

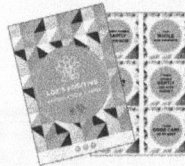

DOWNLOAD YOUR AFFIRMATION CARDS lozlife.com/book-positive

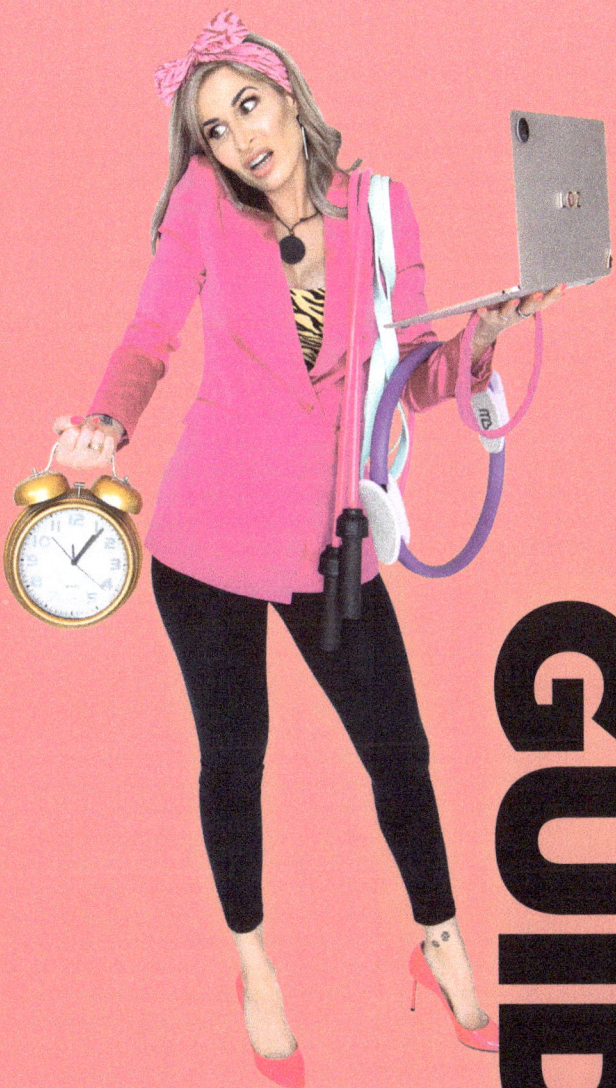

QUICK START GUIDE

Welcome to *Get the F*ck Unstuck!* Congrats on taking the first step in moving from stuck to unstoppable – that is, picking up a copy of my book. Go high five yourself. I'll wait here.

How are you feeling right now? Positive? Overwhelmed? Anxious? Lost? Ready to tackle the book? Need help figuring out where to start?

* Maybe you're feeling okay, but you need a kick up the pants and a dose of motivation.

* Maybe you're eating well, but you need to exercise.

* Perhaps you've lost your momentum.

* Maybe you need to implement healthier eating habits.

I know you're busy, and I realise you may not need all the information in this book right now. Also, while some of you do need it all, you might be feeling a tad swamped with information overload, so eating the elephant one bite at a time might be a more manageable approach.

If you're ready to consume this book from front to back, then get after it! (you can skip this section).

However, if you're looking for speedy guidance or fast access to tools you can use to assist with a specific issue today, this Quick Start Guide will help. All you need to do is read over the following statements and questions, see what resonates with you, and head directly to the relevant page (and Loz Lesson). Yes, it's a solution fast track!

➡ "I'm so stuck I don't even know what's wrong in my life." – head to page 30 (Wellness Assessment)

➡ "I feel stuck in my life and have lost momentum." – head to page 59 (Momentum)

➡ "I need to kick my unhealthy habits to the curb." – head to page 51 (What is the Relationship Between Goals and Habits?)

➡ "I desperately want to build healthy habits when it comes to what I eat." – head to page 107 (The New Food Pyramid)

➡ "I need to move more, and I don't know where or how to start!" – head to page 175 (Movement)

➡ "I have lost my sense of purpose." – head to page 170 (Is Your Mindset Holding You Back?)

➡ "I care too much about what others think." – head to page 77 (My Top Tips to Create Momentum)

➡ "I have trouble sleeping." – head to page 143 (Sleep is What Dreams Are Made of)

➡ "I am so tired all of the time." – head to page 101 (Do You Feel Tired a Lot of the Time?)

➡ "How do I reduce the overwhelm I feel every day?" – head to page 68 (Loz Lesson – Mindset Map)

➡ "How can I live a more mindful life?" – head to page 162 (How Can I Start Practising Mindfulness?)

➡ "What's the best food for me to eat?" – head to page 107 (The New Food Pyramid)

➡ "I need to lose weight urgently." – head to page 99 (Menu)

It's Okay to Feel Stuck

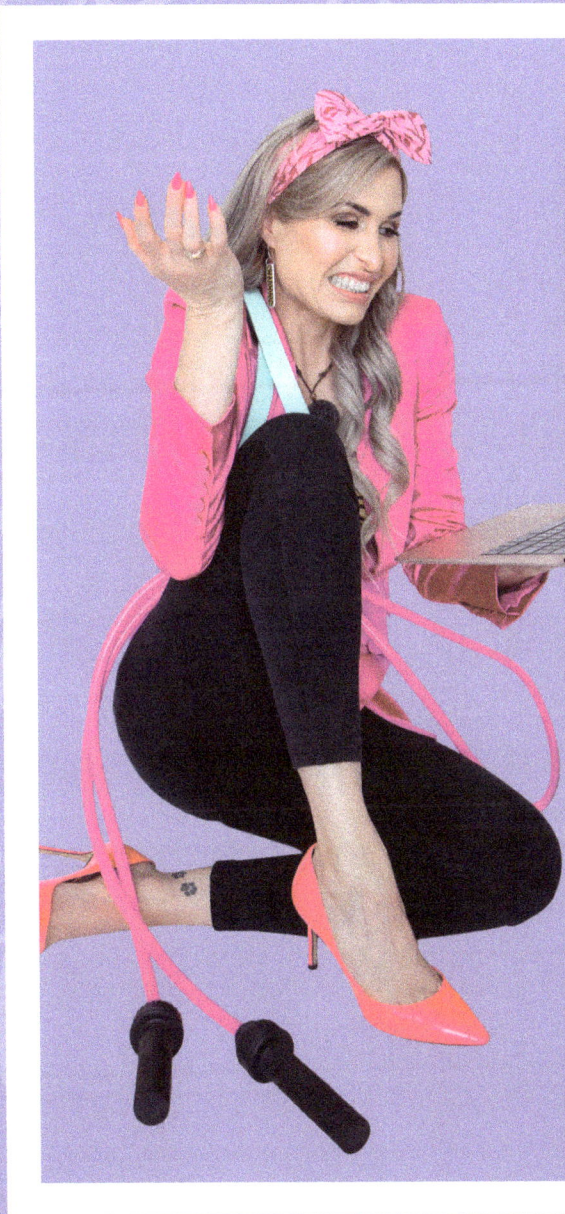

THE POWER OF YOU

A lot of people come to see me because they're feeling really stuck and are not sure how or where to start to make positive changes to get the life they want.

They'll often say things like, "I don't like where I am in my life," "I feel like I haven't really achieved what I thought I would have achieved by now," or, "I'm always tired, and I'm really stressed all the time." Sound familiar?

Do you ever wish you had more energy and could jump out of bed every day, ready to kick some goals, but you're a bit stumped about your first step?

It all starts with an honest conversation!

Start conversing with yourself to see where you're at and, more importantly, where you *want* to be. Is your weight a concern to you? Do you feel like, *I'm overweight, and summer is coming, and I want to be able to do more with the kids? I want to be able to wear shorts. I want more energy so I'm not craving sugar by 3 pm every afternoon to get through the day.*

This is where momentum comes in. It's about taking one small step while simultaneously improving one thing to get the ball rolling.

What handbrakes are holding you back?

Imagine you're driving a car that has five handbrakes on. A car with the handbrake engaged can still move. It's not optimal. It groans and resists, lurching forward reluctantly. But, when you finally remember to release the handbrake, the change is immediate, and all at once you feel like you can do anything and go anywhere because you've gained momentum. Human beings work the same way. We're too often held back by Handbrake Habits. If we can unlock just one of those, you'll find that your life begins to move. It'll still be slow, but it will start to gain some momentum. And the more speed you get by making small changes – breathing better, moving more, drinking more water – the more you'll find the other handbrakes start to get unstuck, so you begin to move faster and more efficiently.

It's about focusing on the one thing that will give you the most significant impact and then committing to doing that one thing first.

Meet yourself where you are right now.

Look at the five healthy habits you're already doing – breathing, sleeping, eating, hydrating, and moving – and see where you can make minor adjustments to set yourself on the path to a healthier, more energised future you.

You could already be doing one or two of them well. You might be getting a great night's sleep, drinking plenty of water, and eating reasonably healthy meals, but you're getting frustrated because you're not feeling or looking any different. Those are probably not the biggest handbrakes holding you back. You may need to remember to get up and move when you sit at your desk all day. Or how you're sitting and looking at your screen may be preventing you from breathing correctly, which means your body and brain are not getting the oxygen they need. So, as a result, you feel foggy or cloudy. And many people 'fix' that fogginess by having coffee, sugar, alcohol, or tobacco.

So, one small change could be to get up from your desk regularly and check that your breathing is nice and deep. See how much clearer your brain feels once you start doing this, and you may find you're not reaching for the 3 pm chocolate fix.

And, just like that, you've released one of the handbrakes holding you back. But that's just one example. Throughout this book, we'll identify the exact handbrakes that are keeping you stuck in place and release them with new, healthy habits.

DON'T FEEL GUILTY ABOUT INVESTING IN YOURSELF

Does the thought of investing in yourself, either with time or money, make you worry that you're being selfish? Do you think about all the other things you should be doing and buying for other people, constantly putting yourself and your needs in last place? While this can be a familiar feeling for many, I find women tend to experience more guilt when focusing on their health and wellbeing.

Many women say that although they know they should take some time out for self-care, their kids, partner, work, and home all take priority. Or, in many instances, they feel guilty spending money on themselves that could be used to buy things for the family, worrying that they're taking away from their families to take care of themselves.

The good news is that you can do some super simple things for yourself that won't break the bank or take time away from your commitments. Here are a few easy ones you can start straight away!

Start by asking yourself what you're prepared to change or add to your daily routine.

* Do you need to drink more water? Could you drink just one extra glass of water each day?

* Do you need to eat more veggies? Could you add one more vegetable to dinner tonight?

* Would you be prepared to go for a short walk with the dog around the block every afternoon? It doesn't have to be a fast walk. Maybe 30 minutes a day is too big of a commitment, but what about just 5 or 10 minutes each day?

* Do you have a foggy brain? Instead of eating chocolate at 3 pm, could you get up from your desk every hour for a couple of minutes and move?

* Can you take a moment to check your breathing while you're working? Are you breathing deeply into your diaphragm through your nose, or are you breathing shallowly through your mouth and feeling foggy?

If this is feeling a bit overwhelming, never fear! We're going to break this whole thing down, one step at a time.

STUCK IN THE MUD

When I was a kid, I used to play a game called 'stuck in the mud' with my friends. Maybe you played it, or your kids do. We would all run around the backyard until one of us was tagged (by the 'it' player), and then we were officially 'stuck in the mud' (completely still, arms up, legs apart) until one of our buddies crawled through our legs to set us free.

Magically, we were instantly free to play again. If only becoming 'unstuck' were that easy as an adult. Unfortunately, it's a lot more work, but it can be done.

Sometimes that mud feels more like quicksand. Sometimes you don't just feel stuck; you feel like you're sinking deeper and deeper, and you don't know how to save yourself.

I hear the phrase "I just feel stuck" daily. I get it. It's the reason why I started Loz Life. I love helping people move past feeling stuck to reclaim their lives and achieve their goals.

So, why do so many of us feel stuck? And I say 'us', as I have been there too. I have felt overwhelmed, stuck, lost, and scared. I have self-sabotaged my happiness. I have given in to feelings of guilt and shame, and I have used every excuse in the book for not making the right choices. Sound familiar? I did the work – the hard way – and here I am today. So, how can you move from stuck to unstoppable, getting the f*ck unstuck?

Having a sense of purpose is crucial. When you don't, or you lose it, you may experience an existential crisis – this is the ultimate sense of being stuck!

Deeper meaning and purpose can serve as a compass for life. Your passion for this purpose will motivate you out of 'stuckness'.

Knowing your purpose, or why, is the first step in the Stuck to Unstoppable process.

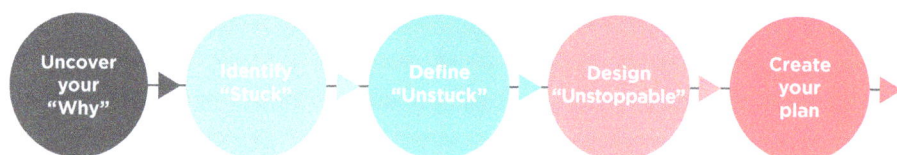

Uncover your "Why" → Identify "Stuck" → Define "Unstuck" → Design "Unstoppable" → Create your plan

Next, you need to identify and own the fact that you are stuck, which can manifest in several ways. When I work with clients, we cover the following in a Wellness Assessment (you can access this in detail on page 30):

* Do you struggle to sleep well?

* Do you feel stressed or overwhelmed?

* Have you gained weight?

* Have you lost a significant amount of weight unplanned?

* Does your diet leave a lot to be desired?

* Do you need more energy?

* Are you able to set and achieve goals?

* Is your self-confidence lacking?

* Do you find it difficult to relax?

* Do you love who you see in the mirror?

We then need to identify where exactly you're stuck, which could be one or many of the following areas in your life:

* Health (physical, mental, emotional)

* Friends and family

* Significant other

* Personal growth

* Fun and leisure

* Home environment

* Career

* Money

Being stuck in one of these areas can quickly flow into others. You might be stuck in a dysfunctional relationship. This can reduce the fun and happiness you have, bring about drama with your family, and cause you to overeat, impacting your health and vitality.

Owning where you are at this exact moment in your life and why you got here is incredibly powerful and empowering. It's the first step in moving from stuck to unstoppable, and, honestly, it's the hardest step.

Next, we will work to define what unstuck looks like for you. What kind of relationship will make you happy and fulfilled? What's the next step you should be taking at work? How can you move, eat, sleep, and recover better for an unstoppable life?

And now to the fun bit – designing your unstoppable dream life and the non-negotiable steps required to achieve it. Unfortunately, too many of us rely on 'hopeium' and wait and hope that our ideal life will just manifest. A solid plan is essential!

So, what are the steps to move from stuck to unstoppable?

1. Uncover and own your why, purpose, values, and beliefs.

2. Identify that you're stuck – where and why.

3. Define what unstuck looks and feels like for you.

4. Design your unstoppable life.

5. Create a plan, and crush it!

Over the years, I've been helping people, just like you, move from stuck to unstoppable. I've worked out that we all fall into one of three Wellness Continuum zones. Based on the patterns of the hundreds of clients I've worked with, I've classified 'stuck', 'unstuck', and 'unstoppable' into defined sets of symptoms, and, to be honest, most people's 'stuck' looks quite similar and sits under the label of 'noticeable signs of cellular stress'.

The three distinct stages of The Wellness Continuum are easy to transition to once you work through the Stuck to Unstoppable process.

Moving from stuck to unstuck is a simple case of enhancing your daily routine by focusing on the Handbrake Habit that's keeping you the most stuck. Remember, this will be eating, breathing, sleep, movement, or hydration.

Once we have released one of those habits, chances are you'll have incidentally released at least one more and will be feeling a hell of a lot better! This is when we start to achieve 'good health' and begin to notice that we are feeling unstuck.

For most people, simply becoming unstuck is a big deal. When we can achieve good health, many of us are comfortable hanging out in this zone for a while. Focusing on daily healthy habits makes it possible to maintain a sustainable lifestyle where we feel pretty darned good most of the time. This is usually a giant step, but, once you make it, it will ultimately provide you with the most significant impact on your wellbeing.

Now, you don't have to strive for 'unstoppable' immediately. I prefer people to hone an unstuck lifestyle until their habits are so automatic that they become their new normal. Moving from unstuck to unstoppable is a much more subtle transition and can only be actioned once your daily healthy habits are solidified in your routine.

Moving to the performance and bio-optimisation zone is about taking those healthy habits and tweaking them, 1 percent at a time, to gain the edge to live an unstoppable life where your imagination becomes the only limiting factor. At this stage in the Wellness Continuum, many clients will work with me to deepen their understanding of mind and body mechanics to uncover subtle hacks for further optimisation. We may use supplements, wearable devices, and other forms of transformative technology to incrementally shift that wellness needle towards peak performance. I'm not going to lie – this part of the process excites me the most because I understand the powerful impact of these seemingly tiny tweaks.

Noticeable Signs
of Cellular Stress

Achievement of
"Good Health"

Performance &
Bio-Optimisation

Stuck

Unstuck

Unstoppable

Routine
Improvement

Habit
Optimisation

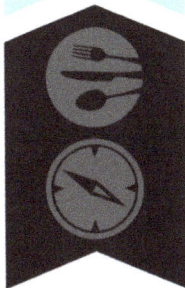

- Medicated/Get Sick Easily
- Inflammation or Pain
- Poor Sleep or Tiredness
- Stressed/Self-Sabotage
- Weight Gain/Loss
- A Sense of Overwhelm/Guilt
- Low Energy or Motivation
- Digestive Issues

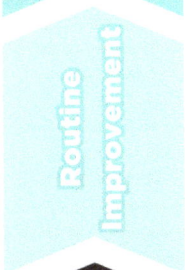

- Moving With More Ease
- Feeling In Control of Eating
- Waking Up Feeling Energised
- Bouncing Back Better
- Improved Body Confidence
- Thinking With Clarity
- Feeling Less Stressed
- Improved Daily Routine

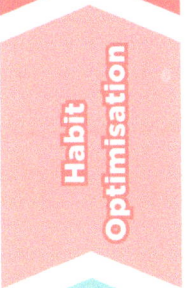

- Energy To Do What You Love
- A Sense of Freedom
- Intuitive Body Awareness
- Moving & Thinking Mindfully
- Confidence To Perform
- Practicing Self-Kindness
- Collectively Conscious
- Actively Seeking Challenge

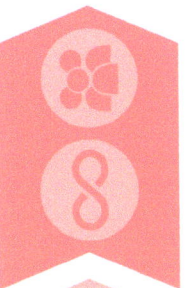

WELLNESS ASSESSMENT

You can use my Wellness Assessment to help you start to unpack your daily routine and identify where you might be most stuck.

Questions about You

In your current roles (in business and life), how many people a day would you say you support/lead/cheer on/lift?

◇ 1–5

◇ 6–10

◇ 11–25

◇ 26+

How do you fill your cup?

_____

_____

_____

_____

_____

Body Metrics

Height _____   *Current body weight* _____

Waist circumference _____   *Ideal body weight* _____

How are you connected to this ideal body weight number? (for example, was this weight before kids, or did you feel strong and healthy at this weight?)

_____

_____

_____

Physical Activity

Current Daily Activity

◇ Sedentary – Sitting at the computer most of the day, or sitting at a desk

◇ Lightly active – Light industrial work, sales or office work that comprises light activities

◇ Moderately active – On your feet, comprised of moderate activity (for example, cleaning, kitchen staff, or delivering mail on foot or by bicycle)

Current Workout Activity

◇ Sedentary – No working out

◇ Lightly active – Low-intensity aerobics

◇ Moderately active – High-intensity aerobics or weight training

◇ Very active – Weights 3+ days per week and aerobics

◇ Extremely active – 2+ hours per day and athletes

Goals

Here is a list of possible goals:

◇ Lose fat
◇ Gain weight
◇ Maintain weight
◇ Add muscle
◇ Improve physical fitness
◇ Look better
◇ Feel better
◇ Have more energy/vitality
◇ Get control of eating habits
◇ Get stronger
◇ Create better balance
◇ Feel less stressed
◇ Love me more
◇ Sleep better
◇ Something else

In general, what are your goals? Write down all the goals from above that apply.

_____

_____

_____

_____

_____

_____

Please list all of your concerns about your health, eating habits, fitness, and body.

_____

_____

_____

_____

_____

_____

Out of those concerns listed, which ones feel most important or urgent?

_____

_____

_____

_____

What makes them important or urgent to you?

_____

_____

_____

_____

What support would you expect from a coach or mentor?

_____

_____

_____

_____

Motivation and Support

What are your top three priorities in life?

_____

_____

_____

How would you like your lifestyle and wellness to be different?

_____

_____

_____

_____

_____

_____

_____

On a scale of 1 to 10, with 1 = not willing at all and 10 = extremely willing, how willing are you to significantly modify your diet?

_____

On a scale of 1 to 10, with 1 = not willing at all and 10 = extremely willing, how willing are you to engage in regular exercise/activity?

_____

How many days would be ideal for participating in a structured movement program?
◇ Ad hoc because I don't have a consistent schedule
◇ 2 days per week
◇ 3 days per week
◇ 4 days per week
◇ 5 days per week
◇ 6 days per week
◇ 7 days per week

On a scale of 1 to 10, with 1 = not willing at all and 10 = extremely willing, how willing are you to keep a record of dietary intake, physical activity, and weight?

_____

On a scale of 1 to 10, with 1 = not willing at all and 10 = extremely willing, how willing are you to alter your work and home environment (for example, remove or reduce accessibility to treats in the kitchen or at your desk)?

_____

On a scale of 1 to 10, with 1 = not willing at all and 10 = extremely willing, how willing are you to practise relaxation techniques regularly?

_____

On a scale of 1 to 10, with 1 = not willing at all and 10 = extremely willing, how ready are you to improve your sleep habits?

_____

On a scale of 1 to 10, with 1 = not willing at all and 10 = extremely willing, how ready are you to take nutritional or herbal supplements each day?

_____

On a scale of 1 to 10, with 1 = not willing at all and 10 = extremely willing, how willing are you to connect with a coach regularly to assess your progress?

_____

With guidance and support, on a scale of 1 to 10, with 1 = not confident at all and 10 = extremely confident, how confident are you in following through on the above activities?

_____

What challenges do you anticipate will impact your journey to creating sustainable wellness (for example, long work hours, lack of social support, childcare, motivation)?

_____

_____

_____

_____

Is anyone else involved in your decision-making regarding how you choose to improve your lifestyle? If so, please briefly detail.

_____

_____

_____

How do you feel about yourself when you're alone?

_____

_____

_____

_____

What is something about yourself you believe is true but probably isn't?

_____

_____

_____

Past Results

What is your previous training experience? Please write 'none' if you have not trained before.

_____

_____

_____

_____

Have you worked with a coach before? If so, when?

_____

_____

_____

Have you tried anything in the past to change your habits, health, eating, and your body? If so, what?

_____

_____

_____

Which of those things worked well for you (even if you might not be doing them now)?

_____

_____

_____

Which of those things did not work well for you?

_____

_____

_____

If you could improve your health in three ways, what would they be?

_____

_____

_____

Health

On a scale of 1 to 10, with 1 = horrible and 10 = awesome, how do you rank your health right now?

_____

Why?

_____

_____

_____

_____

Using the same scale, how would you rate your energy levels?

_____

What's your current energy goal?

_____

_____

_____

_____

Daily Routine

What time do you go to bed?

_____

Do you fall asleep straight away or does it take a while?

_____

What time do you wake up?

_____

Do you wake at the same time each day, even when you're on holidays?

_____

Do you wake up with any of the following?
◇ Fatigue
◇ Dry mouth
◇ Headache
◇ The feeling that you don't want to get up
◇ Pain in your body

What time do you first eat or drink something once you've woken up?

_____

What do you typically have for breakfast?

_____

_____

_____

_____

What do you typically have for a midmorning snack?

_____

What time do you normally have this snack (if not applicable, write n/a)?

_____

What do you typically have for lunch?

_____

_____

_____

_____

What time do you normally eat lunch?

_____

What do you typically have for a midafternoon snack (if not applicable, write N/A)?

_____

What time do you normally have this snack?

_____

What do you typically have for dinner?

_____

_____

_____

What time do you normally eat dinner?

_____

If you have dessert, what would it typically be?

_____

How much water do you drink each day?

◇ Less than 1 L   ◇ I wouldn't say I like water
◇ 1–2 L   and I prefer to drink other
◇ 2–4 L   stuff
◇ More than 4 L

Do you like the idea of following a meal plan to help you stay accountable for your daily food intake?

_____

Do you like the idea of using a mobile app to scan food barcodes and log your food intake manually to help you stay accountable about what you eat?

_____

On a scale of 1 to 10, with 1 = chilled and 10 = very stressed, how would you rate your stress levels?

_____

Discretionary Choices

What are your vices? Choose all that apply:

◇ Chocolate   ◇ Sugary beverages

◇ Chips/crisps   ◇ Caffeine

◇ Alcohol   ◇ Other

◇ Fast food/takeaway

If you drink coffee, how do you have it, and how many do you have per day?

_____

How much do you typically spend on breakfast, lunch, coffee/soft drinks, and vices DAILY?

◇ $1–5

◇ $5–10

◇ $10–15

◇ $15–20

◇ $20+

Commitment

On a scale of 1 to 10, with 1 = I'm not and 10 = I'm all-in!, how committed are you to yourself and change?

_____

Once you've completed the Wellness Assessment, you'll have a much clearer idea of where you are, where you want to go, and what you're willing to do to get there. Do you want to know the best part? Your journey has already begun!

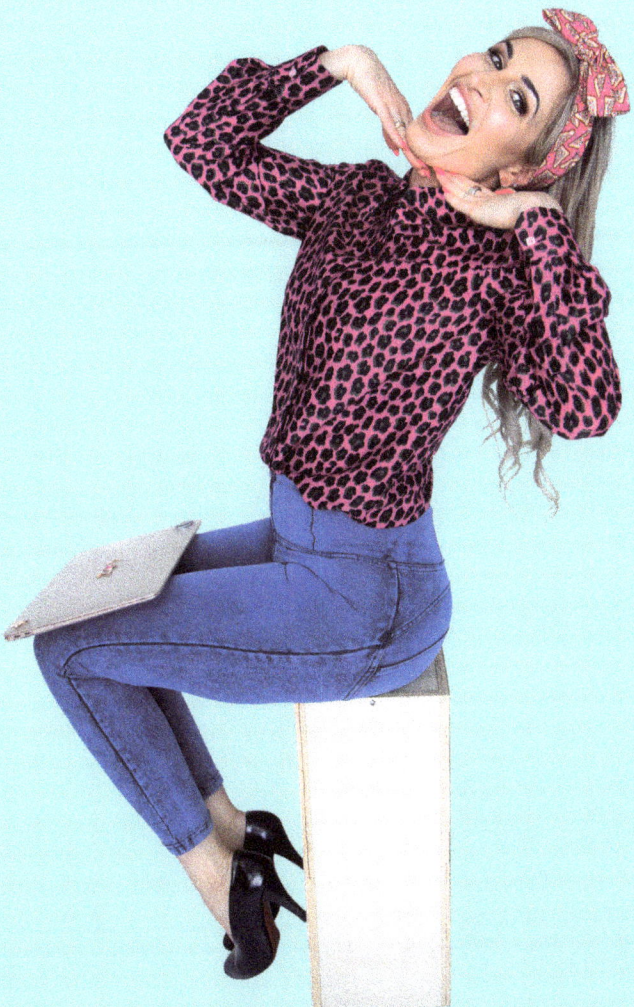

THE BASICS

MY SIX TIPS FOR SETTING ACHIEVABLE GOALS

Setting goals is one thing, but setting realistic, *achievable* goals is the key to getting to where you want to go. When it comes to setting goals, certain strategies work better than others. Luckily, over time, I've learnt what works and what doesn't so you don't have to bother with all the tedious trial and error. The following tips will have you goal setting like a pro in no time.

1. Know your why

But *why*? When you set goals, they must be motivating and align with your highest values. Define them, ensuring they are important and have meaning when accomplished. If there is little to no interest in the outcome, or getting to the end goal seems irrelevant, you will likely have no interest in working towards making it happen. So, why do you want to achieve your goal? How will it change your life? Focus on your why, as it will help you stay motivated.

2. Motivation and momentum are vital to achieving your goals

You need to set your focus on prioritising your goals. Remember – fewer, bigger, better! Too many goals will leave you with little time or energy to achieve them. It would be best if you were committed to enabling success and placing a sense of urgency on your goals. If you fail to prioritise, you could end up putting off the strategic steps required for the end goal to come to fruition. Lack of focus will eventually leave you feeling disappointed and frustrated with yourself, which can be demotivating, and you'll achieve a whole lot of very little. Focus is da bomb.

3. Be SMART

Getting smart about goal setting is a real thing! For goals to be compelling, they need to be smart.

To be smart, you need to apply the SMART rule. With many variations out there, the main message is that goals need to be:

➡ **S**pecific

➡ **M**easurable

➡ **A**ttainable

➡ **R**elevant

➡ **T**imely

Specific

Set yourself a well-defined and focused goal that's as specific as possible. Setting a goal to 'lose weight', for example, doesn't detail enough information to make it achievable because it's vague and quite generalised. Subsequently, you'll end up losing clear direction. What does 'lose weight' mean? How much weight do you want to lose? Goals need specific direction to show you the path. For example, "I want to lose 10 kilos." Be specific about where you are heading and where you want your goal to take you. Focus on the result, and your why.

Measurable

Create measures against your goals, such as dates or amounts, to allow you to measure your success. If your goal is to 'lower expenses', how do you measure it? By how many dollars a week? Make it measurable by putting a value to it to acknowledge milestones as you achieve them. If you can't measure it, you can't achieve it.

Attainable

Ensure that your goals are attainable without making them too easy. It's a delicate balance. Attaining goals too quickly means you probably need to create some more challenging goals. You don't want to get bored! When you find the right balance, you'll feel like you're frequently levelling up, which generates a strong sense of personal satisfaction.

Relevant

You must ensure your goals are relevant to what you want to achieve long-term. Aligning your goals with your purpose will help you become sharply focused on achieving them, and relevance to a long-term desired outcome will help you understand what you need to do to reach your destination. If a goal is not relevant to what you want to achieve, replace it with something that is. Don't set yourself a certain goal simply because everyone else is doing it. Make it relevant to *you*.

Timely

There has to be a time line with a deadline clearly marked. Creating an appropriate and timely goal will assist with the drive and urgency to achieve it. A great example would be a goal of, "I want to lose 10 kilos by the beginning of summer because I want to feel energetic and look fit and healthy on the beach."

4. Get writing

If you're anything like the person I used to be, you love having ideas rolling around in your head. They make sense there. Previously, I believed I could reach my goals simply by thinking about them a lot. The truth is, that thought pattern never really worked for me. I would find myself doing heaps of tiny things that weren't helping me achieve the big-picture goals I had in my head, keeping me caught in a constant state of 'busy'.

Writing down a goal you want to achieve gives it a sense of realism. Once it's translated from head to paper, it's much harder to forget, or deny. So, kinaesthetically transcribing your goal into written words will indirectly help you focus on achieving it. Funnily enough, as soon as I started using an old-school diary again (I hadn't used one since high school), I started achieving *all* of my goals. True story. I love writing actual words on paper with a pen. It's super cathartic and powerful.

My tip

Rather than having a to-do list, create a success list and write goals and tasks using positive language, starting with "I will."

Once written down, place your goals somewhere you can see them regularly to remind you what they are. Post-it notes are a great way to keep tabs on your intentions! I place them all around my office and home where I can see them. They keep me inspired and accountable.

Another method is to start a journal where you keep track of everything. Write down what has worked and what has not and why you think your feelings might be what they are.

For journalling (aka writing shit down), here are a few ideas:

* Write your **top five goals** and list why each is important.

* Write how you want to **feel** after achieving each of them and why you would feel this way.

* Write down the **indicators** that will help you realise when you have reached each goal.

* Write down what **support** you believe you will need to achieve your goal.

* Write down your **celebration list** – those milestones you will hit along the way to encourage you to continue towards your goal. Celebration is key.

5. Start actioning

Remember, a goal is a dream if you don't have a plan. Plans require action to get anywhere. If you've set a meaningful goal and are serious about smashing it, you need to start actioning your plan to get it done. Plan every step of the way, as small as each step may be. Measure your success and celebrate your wins. Be focused. As you complete each item on your success list, cross it off and high five yourself. There's nothing quite as satisfying as looking at your list at the end of a busy day or week and seeing meaningful tasks completed. It's a freaking incredible feeling.

6. Stick to it!

Goal setting is an ongoing task and needs constant reviewing and readjusting. While the end goal may remain the same, the actions that lead you to it can often change. Create reminders on your phone, in your diary and calendar, or use Post-it notes. Don't forget the SMART rules when reviewing your goals and action plan.

These simple strategies will help you set and achieve purposeful goals. So, stay focused as you take yourself on a journey of sustainable growth, abundance, health, and mobility. It's a journey that will set you up for lifelong vitality and help you get the f*ck unstuck, get out of your own way, and achieve your wildest dreams – and then some.

THE POWER OF HEALTHY HABITS

The best way to get unstuck is to create healthy habits. Easy, right? I have morphed my adversities into my most prominent advantages and stopped being average. I have moved through the stages of grief and discovered losing a loved one to be the most poetically cathartic experience I could have ever been gifted. It has taught me how to conquer my deepest fears.

I have genuinely levelled up my life, and I want to share my blueprint for how to do this with you to inspire you to do the same. Because newsflash – you can! How did I achieve this? Simply put, I uncovered the unhealthy habits that kept me stuck in my patterns of destructive thinking and doing. When I worked out that I was living my life by someone else's set of values, I re-evaluated my poor relationship with food, unlocked the power of my life purpose by undertaking daily self-development activities, including mindful meditation, and then started moving my body in a way that felt good and honoured my energetic flow. Luckily for you, I have blueprinted my process and developed the Healthy Habit Hierarchy – a systemised approach to healthy habit stacking for long-term vitality. Hence, this book!

For clarity, let's define a 'habit' as a repetitive behaviour we undertake in a specific context or response to a particular stimulus. Some habits are anchored to an environment – for instance, many people associate 'sleep' with a bedroom. Other habits are situational and may be triggered by a conditioned behavioural bias in certain situations – for example, binge-eating when you feel depressed or bored. Yep, we've all been there. Chocolate is my binge-eating food of choice (I just now prefer dark over milk varieties!).

When we refer to 'unhealthy' habits, these are the behaviours and actions that provide immediate gratification but have long-term negative implications for health – for example, eating doughnuts every day (they taste great when you eat them but if you eat them every day, you'll probably gain weight).

'Healthy' habits may be challenging in the short term but positively impact long-term wellbeing – for example, going to the gym (finding the motivation and energy to exercise can be challenging but if you do it every day, you will gain fitness).

With all the diet, meditation, and exercise trends and options available, it is hard to navigate the best path to living a long and healthy life. I get it. It can be super overwhelming. Are carbs good or evil? What about protein? Sugar? How much is too much? How much should I exercise? Are shakes okay? Should I fast? Eeeeeeek! It's pretty overwhelming, yeah?

A healthy life of freedom cannot be gained by pills, hacks, or shortcuts (aka shakes – sorry, I'm not a fan!). In the end, shortcuts only really provide short-term progress and long-term metabolic confusion. Not the outcome we want.

By following my simple approach to habit improvement, you'll be able to replace your unhealthy habits with revised healthy habits that will be easy to maintain. When you stack these behavioural changes in the most effective order – as per the Healthy Habit Hierarchy – you pave the way for meaningful, lifelong change.

The biggest challenge is that life ebbs and flows, and, for continued success, we must have a sustainable blueprint to follow to self-identify the times we get stuck and to effectively remain unstoppable.

WHAT IS THE RELATIONSHIP BETWEEN GOALS AND HABITS?

The first thing we need to discuss about habits is triggers. A trigger attaches to a habit, and you can take advantage of these to move closer to your goal. They're super powerful. A trigger can be a meal, a particular time of day, or even a room. Once you attach that trigger to making your new healthy habit, it will become easier.

This is where willpower is valuable, and my strategy is to use it first thing in the morning. Upon rising, your will is at its highest. Use this increased willpower to start creating a routine that elevates you so you're not having to draw on your depleted energy in the evening after work. For example, as soon as I wake up, I *do not* check my emails but, instead, spring out of bed. I then complete my ablutions, sit down, and enjoy a five-minute meditation with my coffee to set myself up for success. This primes me to experience the rest of my day from a calm place. I then jump on my rebounder trampoline and undertake a few lower-body warm-up exercises on my Pilates reformer or do some yoga to get my body moving.

When I'm in my peak energetic state, I go for a 10–20-minute walk, rain, hail, or shine! When I return, I make a healthy brekkie and prepare lunch and dinner in advance, which could be my clean spaghetti fauxlognaise (it doesn't have garlic, dairy, or gluten, so I can't call it bolognaise!). This way, I don't have to think about or prepare something to eat when I arrive home from a productive day in the evening.

As you can see, I utilise all the levels in the Healthy Habit Hierarchy by capitalising on my willpower and morning momentum. I follow a pretty similar routine every single day, even when I'm on holiday. People find it strange that I meditate, exercise, and eat healthy on holidays, but all those activities make me feel fantastic. Why wouldn't I want to feel awesome when I'm having a break? Don't you want to feel awesome too?

When you look at it, it's pretty much a case of lining up all the dominoes for the day and knocking down that first one. The rest will take care of themselves. After all, it's routine that helps keep you rolling in the right direction. In no time, new healthy habits will form, and you'll be flying towards that goal. Boom!

THE HANDBRAKE HABITS

Eating, breathing, sleeping, moving, and hydrating – we all do them and without them, we couldn't survive!

The health and wellness industry has a way of overwhelming us by convincing the masses that we must have many super intricate daily rituals to be happy, healthy, and thriving.

If you've got to get the kids ready, get yourself ready, drive to work for your nine-to-five gig, do the school pick-up run, make dinner, and spend time with your loved ones, the following scenario just isn't going to be on your radar.

The Influencer's Guide to Success, Confidence, and Happiness

It would be best if you woke up before sunrise to drink a warm glass of water with turmeric, lemon, and a dash of black pepper before running 5 km in a sweatsuit so you can come home for a cold shower where you will hyperventilate to bring oxygen to your brain. Then, find a comfortable position atop a lofty mountain to sit in the lotus position and allow a gentle breeze to brush your face. Notice the eagle soaring overhead as you reach a state of blissful stillness as you meditate for one hour. Upon returning home, you must do ten handstand push-ups on soft grass (to ground yourself and connect with the earth) while balancing a crystal on your right foot as you say your daily affirmations and listen to binaural beats to synergise your mind and body to energetically manifest your divine future.

This is an entirely fictional scenario, but you get the gist of the sheer madness the internet tries to sell us!

I'm always fascinated by trends that set people up for completely unsustainable habits that take a lot of extra time and effort to implement into a busy life. I'm talking about stuff like having to wake up at 3 am, journalling, drinking some elixir or tonic, fasting, cold showers, ice baths, saunas, and extreme activities, which, for the majority of the population, are either inaccessible or just absolutely never going to fit in the average working person's daily schedule. Now, I'm all for *all* the things I just mentioned because each has some incredible benefits (and, yeah, I do a lot of them myself). Still, when it comes to moving from stuck to unstuck, it's gotta be simple, practical, doable, and repeatable, so why not start with the five Handbrake Habits you're already doing and focus on doing at least one of them better?

What I love about the concept of Handbrake Habits is they all have a relationship with and will indirectly affect each other. For example, if we can enhance our eating, our sleep, hydration, and movement will most likely improve. Likewise, if we can focus on breathing better, our sleep and movement will also benefit.

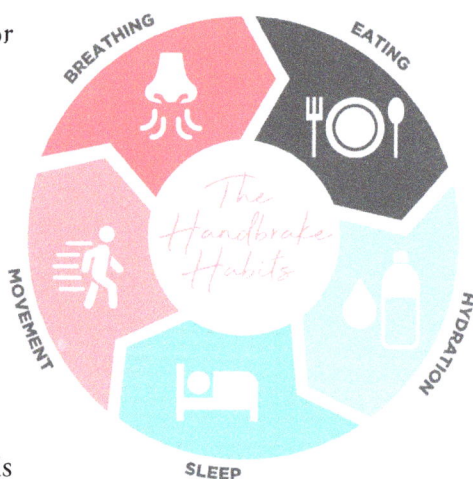

Each of these five habits is weaved within the Healthy Habit Hierarchy and plays a vital role in improving lifelong happiness, health, and vitality when moving from stuck to unstoppable.

Think about the Handbrake Habits as your daily points of focus and the Healthy Habit Hierarchy as your long-term blueprint to live an incredible and inspiring life.

THE HEALTHY HABIT HIERARCHY

What's the Healthy Habit Hierarchy, I hear you ask? Excellent question, and one we will delve into throughout the book, with a chapter dedicated to each step in the hierarchy:

1. Momentum

2. Menu

3. Mindset

4. Movement

5. Mastery

6. Mentorship – a new addition to the hierarchy and the reason for updating my book!

Guide and connect with others to expand the collective consciousness through mentorship
Mentorship

Reprogram and gain mastery for unstoppable performance, focus and confidence
Mastery

Improve your movement and posture for pain free living
Movement

Unlock resilient mindset and bulletproof sleep habits
Mindset

Optimise eating, hydration and breathing
Menu

Identify unstuck for max momentum
Momentum

Establish Momentum

The first step is establishing the momentum you need to move to your new life. We'll start by exploring:

* Where are you in your life?
* Why aren't you there yet?

* Where do you want to be?
* What's getting in your way?

* What are you prepared to change to set your life direction?

Optimise Your Menu

Once the momentum is rolling, you can explore the intakes or inbound things in your life and optimise them. Questions we'll cover here include:

* What are you consuming?

* How's your breathing?

* How much water are you drinking?

* Are you mindful of your daily activities, social circle, and choice of media?

* What's going on with your gut health?

* Do you know your carbohydrate tolerance?

Create a Great Mindset

Now that you're biochemically more optimised, you can learn to find space to quieten your mind, improve sleep, sharpen your focus, and set purposeful and intentional goals.

Improve Your Movement

Regardless of your fitness goals, learn to improve your movement and breathing for increased physical freedom, pain reduction, and sustainable mobility – posture and mobility are key.

* How do you want to be able to move in 10, 20, 30, 40 years and beyond?

Repeat, Improve, and Gain Mastery

Learn how to fall back on this blueprint for lifelong happiness, health, and vitality, no matter what curveballs life throws, and pay it forward to others!

Guidance and Connection via Mentorship

Grow your ability to serve others, upgrade your frequency on your mission for challenge and leadership, and expand the collective consciousness by becoming a mentor.

So, that's the Healthy Habit Hierarchy summarised. Now we're going to explore each element in depth, and, as you now know, it all starts with *momentum*.

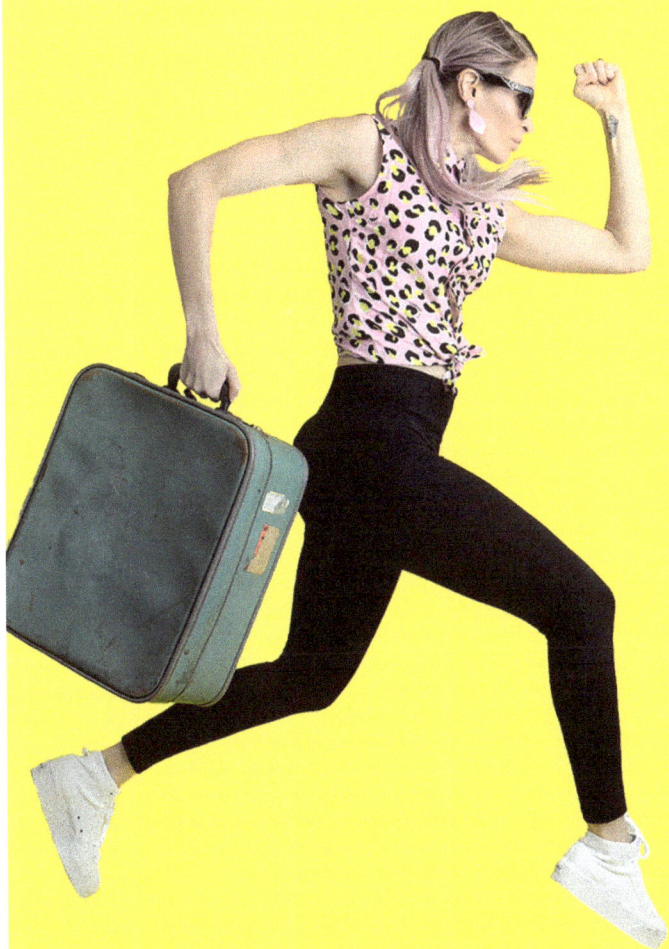

Have you ever felt stuck in your life, your health… even in traffic? That's a yes from me!

I bet there have been times when you've pretended everything was perfect and fabulous, but, on the inside, you were drowning and overwhelmed, right? Chances are you've forgotten the last time you gave yourself a chance to be you. Authentically, unapologetically you.

Do you know who and where you are as you show up daily? Does that person resonate with the person you want to be? Does where you are resonate with where you want to be? So many questions!

Too often, we become obsessed with how we want the world to see us. This is why, for example, apps for enhancing images of our faces exist. And yes, we've all tried it.

I want to run a crazy thought past you. Bear with me.

While we obsess over what people think of us, it's likely that no one is actually judging us; we're all too busy worrying about not looking ridiculous ourselves. If and when people assume things about you, it's a reflection of them, not you. True story.

Sure, I'm not one to point the finger here. Whenever I do so, my husband, Michael, likes to remind me that there are always three pointing back. Since re-evaluating my life and uncovering the unhealthy habits holding me back, I am more conscious than ever about living life on my own terms. And not judging – myself or others.

As workers, partners, parents, and friends, we wear a lot of hats, and we like to create certainty in our lives to keep us comfortable. We plan stuff, add value to the lives of others, and continually hit milestones in our own world – like finding that dream job, getting married, and having a family. We do everything that we feel society tells us will make us good people… good, happy people.

Momentum is the force that drives us, moving us on our current trajectory at the speed of our past, present, and future lives.

It's all about harnessing energy, **because energy is a habit, and its power is freaking remarkable.**

I don't know about you, but sometimes my brain is like a web browser. It's like I have 40 tabs and five windows open at once – and where's that random sound coming from?! But when you start building healthy habits into your life, you'll be able to close down so many of these open tabs, turn off the random annoying sounds, and make your mind feel like a calm web browsing experience.

GETTING STUCK

The problem is, we are so busy being busy, trying to juggle all the things life throws at us – work, family, relationships, health – that, at some point in the chaos, we get stuck. And getting stuck totally *sucks*.

It's when the washing needs doing, dinner needs cooking, your to-do list is the length of the Nile River, the kids are fighting, you haven't slept enough, and you're also supposed to 'adult'! How on earth are you supposed to *not* be stressed and anxious? It's almost impossible.

When we get stuck, the stress sets in; the weight packs on, and our physical and mental health declines. At this point, we start to question our entire existence, subconsciously asking ourselves, *Can I ever be enough?* And then we suddenly get s-t-u-c-k, caught in this cycle of stuckness, where we feel helpless.

This life is here to be lived, and, for some of us, the simple daily experience of just living passes by because we are too focused on achieving power by always chasing more.

It's true what they say: money doesn't buy you happiness. Not having enough of it to get by can undoubtedly cause stress, but having too much isn't a quick happiness fix.

Now let's talk about being busy.

'Busy' has become the norm and the new answer to, "How are you?" I've been guilty of saying it, doing it, and wearing it as a badge of honour.

Strangely, finding strength is just about taking control, making conscious decisions about your life, and sticking to them. That's it. True power is being able to focus on the stuff worth focusing on and realising that life is, or at least can be, a hell of a lot simpler than we want to admit. Sometimes being busy is an excellent excuse for not achieving stuff.

Do you feel like your life is getting on top of you? Does it feel as if your soul's purpose is being buried deeper and deeper beneath the mounting piles of proverbial shit you keep focusing on, things that aren't even adding any real value to your life? Here's the thing: it's never too late to say no.

MY STORY OF 'STUCK'

Home truth for me: the old me was stuck. Very stuck.

So stuck that, for eight years, I was prescribed antidepressants.

So stuck that I then dropped 20 kg because of the mental and physical stress of acquiring an autoimmune disease.

So stuck that I gained 10 kg in six months after being hospitalised and highly medicated.

So stuck that I had a heap of acronyms from medical professionals thrown at me, labelling me this and that and telling me I'd be on medication for the rest of my life.

The facts:

* I've been the victim of domestic violence in several relationships.

* I was sexually assaulted and spent the night in the hospital once paramedics revived me after my drink was spiked during a social outing at age 21.

* I've been diagnosed with a pituitary tumour and was prescribed medication for two years to shrink it.

* I became a widow when my first husband committed suicide two days after my 31st birthday.

* I've been so physically and emotionally exhausted that I've had a mental breakdown and stayed in bed for months. I've had two more episodes of burnout since.

* I've been so low that I've relied on alcohol, sugar, and stimulants to get me through my day to the point of addiction.

* I've hated my body and loathed myself from the depths of my soul so much that I have wanted to opt out of life.

* I was so f*cking *stuck* that I became obsessed with a fear of dying to the point that I had to take medicine for anxiety.

* I caught COVID-19 four times in a single year yet had minimal time to allow my body to heal because I had to keep multiple businesses afloat amid one of the most challenging economic downturns in recent human history.

Seriously, I know that being stuck sucks.

The thing about getting stuck is that unless we know how to unstick ourselves, we tend to stay in one place, digging ourselves deeper into the ground. That's the definition of being stuck... you literally cannot move, like being stuck in the mud!

HOW I GOT UNSTUCK

You know what? My history is not my identity. I've unstuck myself so effectively that I am the fittest and healthiest I've ever been. I've conquered my deepest fears, travelled the world, kicked most of my medications, and even achieved all of this with an undiscovered, literal hole in my heart (which I've subsequently had repaired by a surgical implant – yay for science!).

I'm not telling you all this to toot my own horn. It wasn't easy. I want to show you that it is possible to release yourself from your stagnation. To move through the mud, you have to know how and why.

That, my dear friend, is called *momentum*, and, for many people, it's about uncovering the most challenging answer to the most straightforward question: What's your *why*?

Momentum is that energy that keeps us moving forward, and sometimes it can move us in the wrong direction. The combination of meaningful momentum and a clear plan that bridges the gap between where we are now and where we want to be is all it takes to turn dreams into achievable, measurable goals that can ultimately create joy and long-term fulfilment.

MOVING FORWARD

One day, not so long ago, I realised that unexpected things would always happen.

With that thought, I realised the only control I have is dealing with difficult situations as I meet them on my path. I can't control whether challenges occur, but I can control how I respond.

Through the challenges, I've moved forward with the intent to thrive with courage, humour, and grace. I now live with that purpose-driven, warrior-woman, gonna-save-the-world vibe, and I know I am the queen of my own life because the choice is always mine.

Think about that – it's super empowering. When you realise you have the power, there's no more blaming others!

Since I worked all of this out, being busy is something other than what I want to be associated with. To me now, being busy almost sounds like you're just distracted. Or making an excuse.

Remaining open, activated, and complete can create meaning by connecting us with other beings. These words convey a much more profound and enriching sense of purpose than just being distracted by a lot of stuff because we're so busy being busy.

Yes, I've achieved a truckload of goals throughout my life, but the most enriching part of this journey has been the ability to take a break, take a breath, and take back power in my life by shedding expectations of myself. Don't get me wrong – I love creating opportunities by saying yes. But, lately, I've been saying no, and, *whoa*, it sure feels good! You should totally try it.

As humans living a human experience, it's easy to worry about how the world sees us. So, we pretend everything is fine, even when it feels like our world has stopped turning. Being busy, multitasking and burning the candle at both ends, these actions are robbing you of your real purpose and the ability to focus.

Honestly, it's okay to be stuck. It's even okay to suck at something we don't want to suck at. Life has its ups and downs, after all. The key is to use these experiences to 'fail forward' by maintaining a clear vision of what we want to achieve. When we do this, nothing can hold us back from unlocking our potential.

So, what does failing forward really mean?

Failing forward is understanding that a person must embrace failure as a stepping stone to future success. To fail forward means that you have chosen to value every loss for the lessons learnt and apply those lessons in future efforts, even if those efforts might also result in failure. When you are failing forward, each failure moves you closer to ultimate success.

Are your dreams so obnoxiously passionate that you would feel a little embarrassed if you said them out loud to someone? If not, they need to be!

Luckily for you, simplicity is the key, and complexity is the enemy of the execution of our goals. We've been conditioned to think that getting stuff done is all about motivation and willpower, and, unfortunately, this is just one big lie. I hate to be the bearer of bad news, but we often focus on our fears instead of our goals to motivate us, which is inherently counterproductive. Remember, a goal without a plan is just a dream.

What thoughts get you moving? What goals ignite a spark? What actions fuel your fire and excite you? It all comes back to momentum.

Momentum is the force that drives us, moving us on our current trajectory at the speed of our past, present, and future lives. It's all about harnessing energy because energy is a habit, and its power is freaking remarkable.

How amazing would it feel to make informed decisions about everything you choose to do because you are so in touch with your truth, your values, and your capacity to add value to the world? Imagine waking up with so much energy and zest for life that you want to spread it throughout your life, just like glitter, every day?

That's the power of momentum.

This section will help you unlock the handbrakes on your life and get the ball rolling so you can set sail towards the life you deserve.

Loz Lesson

Before we continue, download and complete **Mindset Map** to help you close some of the open tabs in your brain.

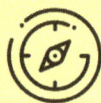

MINDSET MAP

GET IT OUT OF YOUR HEAD

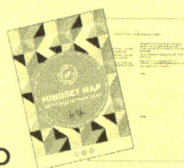

DOWNLOAD YOUR MINDSET MAP **lozlife.com/book-mindset**

WHY ARE YOU STUCK?

Here's a question: What does your ideal life look like, and why? If you could wave a magic wand tomorrow, what would you change? What if you could get the f*ck unstuck?

What actions will you take right now, tomorrow, next week, next month, next year, and every day for the rest of your life to make it happen? What will it look like when you've 'made it'? And why haven't you made it happen already?

In this beautiful life, you only get what you think you deserve. You also get what you focus on. Where focus goes, energy flows.

People who don't have authentic success – that is, the type of success aligned with who they are and who they want to be – tend to believe success is just good luck. The thing is, the harder you work, the luckier you get!

Any successful person will tell you that luck has nothing to do with achievement. In truth, genuine, fulfilling accomplishment sets you apart from the masses. When you smile and project an aura of kindness, warmth, and friendliness out into this big, evil world, you will attract like for like; happiness will be drawn to you. Your vibe attracts your tribe. So, success is about *being* and *owning* the energy you want to attract.

GET BACK TO YOUR ROOTS

Just like natural beauty, peace and love can grow anywhere. It might sound too simple but if you're having difficulty identifying where you're stuck and how you can gain more momentum, remember that living in harmony with nature is essential to nourishing our souls and feeling balanced and joyous in our lives. I always tell people: if your energy is low, get outside. Even if it's cloudy or overcast, just stepping outside can do wonders for your energy levels.

Living in the dark is merely existing. Ten minutes in nature every day can be life-changing. Better still, invest in a red or near infrared light therapy device. I use mine daily to supercharge my vitality!

Your *vibe* attracts your *tribe.*

So, success is about *being* and *owning* the energy you want to attract.

More profoundly, when you nurture nature, nature nurtures you. So, life is all about stepping outside our comfort zones to explore our higher selves. When we go on these paths of discovery, only then can we know where our wild hearts genuinely belong.

Ultimately, you are the greatest masterpiece you will ever have a chance to create. Pretty cool concept, huh? So, why not take your time and make some freaking magic! If you do, the legacy of your life's work will live on, unbounded by the chronological confines of your human experience.

Regarding finding momentum, I've always loved the idea of not being what people expect us to be. I'm quite the social butterfly and find myself at events weekly. My husband calls me a 'seven-day eventist' for laughs. From the outside, people who see me on social media without connecting with my humanness judge me. But I've realised that judgements are just a person's inadequacies projected onto other people.

Next time you feel yourself judging someone, try turning the judgement back on yourself. Why are you judging? What does this judgement say about your own insecurities and fears?

WHAT'S YOUR WHY?

Uncovering your *why* is the best way to deeply connect with your authentic nature. By doing so, you will always prioritise meaningful actions and align them with your highest values. You certainly attract an abundance of inspired people and new opportunities when you sense who you are. Again, like attracts like.

Authenticity is a collection of choices that we have to make every day. It's about the decision to show up and take the opportunity to be honest. It's about letting our true selves show.

Part of my journey has been about following my passion for fitness, wellness, and sustainable vitality. When I competed as a body-sculpting athlete, I'd fall highly ill for months during preps for stage shows. I didn't feel like my usual bubbly self. I couldn't sleep, was burnt out, and my body kept screaming to slow down, but I ignored it all. I kept trying new things to help myself feel better, but, on show days, I was always too lean and not 100 percent myself… and it showed.

Had I listened to my body more during those times when I was ill, I know I could have brought a better physique to the stage. But I didn't, and I have learnt much from that experience. You know what, though? I always rocked my lean little body and had incredible photo shoots before and after my shows! It's all about perspective. I'm super proud of what I achieved.

Because of this experience, I am more aligned and in tune with myself. I'm certainly far more authentic, and I now feel whole, wholesome, and complete, driven to do more than ever. I've allowed every lesson to help shape who I am and propel me to even more exceptional outcomes as I continue to 'be'. Yep, that's failing forward. And, in the words of the great Brené Brown, "daring greatly."

When I thought about how I would explain my ideas on momentum, I asked myself: What information would I have given myself ten years ago? What would have helped me? I'm talking about the if I knew then what I know now, 'how-could-I-have-been-as -big-as-Tony-Robbins-already?' kind of stuff.

To me, turning my life around has been about asking better questions. I am the first to admit that I used to ask terrible questions like, "Why am I fat?", "Why is everyone mean?", "What's wrong with me?", and "Will I ever be enough?"

Honestly, I didn't even ask questions; I assumed my beliefs to be facts. This was my most significant boo-boo. As soon as I started asking myself questions such as, "What can I do to lose weight?", "What parts of myself am I comparing to other people?", "How can I improve myself more?", and "How do I ask better questions?", I was able to strategise actionable steps to uncover the real reasons why I was stuck and could, therefore, do something about it.

As soon as I stepped into my truth and 'got real', I could finally move forward with my life and get onto the momentum train.

If you want to design the life of your dreams, you must first identify how you envision your life in the future.

Loz Lesson

Download and complete **Goal Setting**
and start thinking about where you'd like to be.

GOAL SETTING
LONG TERM GOALS

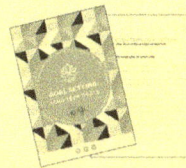

DOWNLOAD YOUR GOAL SETTING **lozlife.com/book-goals**

FORWARD FAILS

At this point, I'd like to talk about some of the forward fails I made and identify the key struggles that slowed me down:

* Trying to out-exercise a bad diet.

* Burning the candle at both ends because being busy and productive was the new normal.

* Attempting every single health craze I'd heard about and then hating myself because I really couldn't commit to them and was, therefore, a hopeless failure, doomed for ill health in old age.

After failing forward for over 20 years, I finally worked out that:

* Wealth is useless without health.

* It's the intangibles, not the tangibles, of life that actually fulfil us.

* The only thing you can control is how you perceive a circumstance or event.

* Where you are right now in your life is a direct by-product of your daily habits, choices, and beliefs.

CLIENT STORY
– CREATING MOMENTUM

Working as a personal trainer (PT) within a gym, I have spent countless hours helping potential clients unpack their challenges, identify where they're stuck, and define what 'unstuck' looks like so they can start creating momentum.

Dave, a lovely gym goer, was struggling to balance family life and work. After giving birth to their third child, Dave's wife decided to focus on looking after their small children while Dave kept the money coming in as a FIFO worker in the mines. With living expenses soaring, he had been feeling the pressure to work longer hours but was finding his energy had decreased significantly since he ramped up his workload.

At 31 years old, he felt he had aged beyond his years in recent months and had developed lower back pain, so he was drinking too much because he found it difficult to wind down when he got home. He decided to start coming to the gym on a casual basis when he was back in town to help improve his fitness. This is how we met.

Dave thought it would be good to chat to a PT (me) because the gym suggested it might help him with his goals. He booked a discovery call and completed my Wellness Assessment – a comprehensive survey that asks people various questions about their lifestyle, their daily routine, their goals, and their obstacles.

Throughout our chat, it was clear that Dave was very stuck. He felt helpless and locked into a FIFO lifestyle because, on one hand, the money was great, but, on the other, he really felt like he was drowning in his poor habits. He realised that he was absorbing a lot of toxic energy from the culture of his colleagues and had developed poor coping mechanisms that led him to self-soothe with alcohol. On top of that, he was drinking six cups of coffee a day and not a lot of water, consequently leading to broken sleep, fatigue upon waking, and very little energy to do much else other than work. Essentially, he had engineered a very unsustainable lifestyle and felt trapped by 'golden handcuffs' because he was making a good wage to support his young family.

By asking Dave some simple questions that elicited responses he had never previously considered, we were able to identify that his daily actions certainly were misaligned with his values – family, security, and personal health. Although he was making money to provide security for his loved ones, it was at the cost of his other two key values. We found some gaps in Dave's daily habit stack where he could make some simple adjustments to satisfy his values of personal health and family. We borrowed time from his 'boys time' in the afternoons and freed up space for Dave to go for a daily walk and catch up with his family on a video call every day while he walked.

When I checked in with Dave a month later, just by making a seemingly small change, he had made the bold decision to overhaul his shifts and take more frequent trips back home so he could spend more time with his family. Funnily enough, five months down the track, he quit his job, attracted an even better job closer to home, and really took the time to work on his personal health. He gave up drinking altogether, joined the gym as a regular member, hired a PT, and got his life back on track. One simple change can be the catalyst for an entire lifestyle transformation.

MY TOP TIPS TO CREATE MOMENTUM

Now, the moment you've been waiting for – here are my top tips for creating the momentum you deserve.

1. Practise makes progress

It is not fear that stops you from doing the brave and 'right' things in your daily life. Instead, the problem is avoidance. Think back to all those things you've held off doing and pushed under the rug. I bet you have a few, huh?

As humans, we want to feel comfortable, so we avoid doing or saying anything that will evoke fear or other challenging emotions. We tend to avoid discomfort. Avoidance will make you feel less vulnerable in the short term, but it will never make you feel less afraid. True story.

We may believe that anxiety and fear don't concern us because we avoid experiencing them. We may keep the scope of our lives narrow and familiar, opting for sameness and safety. We may not even realise that we are scared of success, failure, rejection, criticism, conflict, competition, intimacy, or adventure because we rarely test the limits of our competence and creativity. We avoid anxiety by avoiding risk and change. I can certainly attest to having done this for most of my adult life, and I know I'm not alone.

My tip

Always choose fearless authenticity over everything else. Aligning your actions to your highest-priority values starts in the heart. Each day, we are invited to be who we are and to kick butt!

It's important not to let the desire for perfection get in the way of possible progress.

I believe in embracing our imperfections because that's where the beauty lies.

Sucking at something multiple times is an integral part of development. When a child is learning to walk, you don't just let them sit on the floor, a defeated, crying mess, when they fail on their first attempt, right? No. We encourage them to get back up and try again. This fundamental lesson we learn as toddlers is still incredibly relevant to adulthood – keep practising, and you'll eventually break through! Or, as Dory says, "Just keep swimming."

2. Stop worrying about what other people think

Other people will always judge you, but, frankly, other people's opinions are none of your business. Caring about what other people think is robbing you of your potential momentum. Now is the perfect time to stop watching other people's views because they perpetually prevent you from becoming your best self. Harnessing the power of not giving a f*ck what other people think is life-changing.

Do you know what fear stands for? False evidence appearing real. The thing about fear is that it pretty much drives everything we do.

Truth be told, there are only three things we fear in life (besides snakes, spiders, and other bitey things), and they are:

1.   Success

2.   Failure

3.   Judgement

That. Is. It.

So, this is where it gets tricky. You will experience all of these things at some point in your life. This world is not a jungle. It's more like a human zoo, and you either fight or run (yep, it's the old 'fight or flight' survival instinct). Some days you tame the tiger, and other days the tiger eats you for lunch.

But it is okay to be scared; sometimes, it just means you are about to do something courageous. It's just a matter of understanding that courage is not the absence of fear but the triumph over it. Feel the fear and do it anyway, and all that.

Be the beast that earns its stripes because it's better to live one year as a tiger than a hundred years as a sheep. Know what you want, and don't be afraid to get it.

When someone comes to me saying they suffer from anxiety, I always ask: Who are you trying to please?

It's time to stop worrying about what 'they' may think and learn to live your life authentically… with no f*cks given. Stand tall like a mountain but stay grounded like an oak tree. If you can do this, you will reach great heights by allowing yourself to become shaped by resilience.

In life, a healthy and positive self-image is the best possible preparation we can give ourselves for success. Believe in yourself. Even if you don't right now – and this might sound crazy – pretend that you do because, at some point, you eventually will.

When I first decided to compete in a bodybuilding show that involved wearing a bikini, I found the prospect extremely confronting. You get it. As someone who hated her body, I didn't own a bikini or a one-piece swimsuit. After my first show, however, I fell in love with the process of bodybuilding. It gave me space to connect and surround myself with those fantastic (and crazy) humans who inspire me.

I've found that the sport of bodybuilding seems to attract a particular type of person. The funny thing is that we all understand each other in that specific niche culture. We are driven to do our best for many reasons, but, at the heart of it, we all choose to do something quite extraordinary by asking to be judged on our appearance. It takes immense courage to get up on stage and be judged on your appearance by a panel of strangers, with absolutely no regard for the sacrifices you made to get there. To the outside world, this subculture can appear very superficial. I get it. But, having been in the thick of it, the more open and authentic I am on stage and in my preparation to get there, the more I empower myself for life in general. Consequently, the more I attract equally empowered people into my circle. You only attract who you think you deserve, remember? And you become who you hang around. So, who are you spending your time with these days?

Obviously, I'm not recommending that everyone follow the same route and decide to compete in a bodybuilding competition! Hell no. I recommend you find daily activities where you can regularly step outside your comfort zone – the flow-on effect is incredible. Realistically, most people will never be confident to try something this challenging because we are all scared of rejection to some degree. Again, that's the human experience. However, the reality is that today is the day you can choose to throw away the mask and wear your soul. Or not. But it's your decision.

We must go on adventures to find where we truly belong. Sometimes it feels great to be lost or heading in the wrong direction because we may discover a route to something even more significant.

Remember, life is about the journey, not the destination. Corny but stinking true.

For me, bodybuilding was one of those journeys that unlocked a stack of opportunities I would have otherwise missed had I not chosen to step outside my comfort zone and wear a tiny bikini on stage.

Nobody trips over a mountain. It's the pebbles that cause you to stumble, the things people think are totally irrelevant to your goals. Pass all the stones in your path, and you will eventually find you have crossed the mountain. You have nothing to lose and a whole world to see.

Remember… life is either a daring adventure or nothing at all!

3. Leave comparison behind

Comparison is the death of joy and the end of pleasure. *End of story*. We too often compare our beginnings with someone else's middle.

When I started out in business, if a competitor retailer opened up nearby, I'd go hell for leather to try to outdo them. I'd send in secret shoppers and then stress over how much income this competitor was 'stealing' from me. Consequently, I'd spend heaps of money on marketing only to go over budget and not get anywhere. It was a vicious cycle. Now I realise this action was driven by comparison, inspired by fear.

Having started competing as a bikini fitness model in my 30s, I was much older than many competitors. My first coach reminded me to "stick to my lane" and focus on my ability by playing to my strengths. This simple advice has resonated with me ever since by profoundly shifting my perception of self-worth. I'm now inspired instead of intimidated by my fellow competitors.

Start making *your own rules.*

The sooner you live a life true to *yourself***, the more confidence you will attract, and the more confident you will become.**

It's such a wonderful feeling to let go of comparison. It's possible for you to love the person you are without comparing yourself to anyone else. It's still okay to want to be better than you were yesterday but if you're people-pleasing, that hides the real you. Own who you are, and you will be unstoppable.

Remember, confidence will make you happier and is more sustainable than any diet or shiny, new distraction. How can anyone see how amazing you are if you cannot see it yourself because you're clouded by the shadows you allow others to cast over your radiance? You're freaking awesome!

Over the past few years, since my first husband died, my circle of friends has undergone a complete restructuring. My vibration has shifted dramatically, and, as a result, I have now attracted some incredible new people into my world.

Through this journey, I have learnt that people come into our lives for various reasons. Our lives and our perception of ourselves shift and evolve; it's important to remember that our environment also needs to change to foster our personal development. A new friendship can bring so much mutual value, and it can start with something as simple as a friendly "hello."

I've noticed that people can be antisocial, and I'm pretty sure it's not deliberate. Instead, the fear of being judged seems to impact us all differently. People spend a lot of time worrying about stuff like, "I could never be as successful as…" or, "I could never make as much money as…" or, "I could never be as beautiful as…", and this gets in the way of making quality connections with others. Stupid fear.

When we compare our unique journey to another's, we distract ourselves from the actual comparison. Instead, wouldn't it feel a whole lot more wonderful to be captivated by the inspiration of others to help you find your purpose? Yep.

It's time to give up being embarrassed about who you are and beating yourself up about how others perceive you. People will judge you no matter what, so the less you give a damn, the happier you will ultimately be. In the end, the inauthentic people have an image to maintain. Real people don't have to care. Stop asking permission to break free of the toxicity of the world. Start making your own rules. The sooner you live a life true to yourself, the more confidence you will attract, and the more confident you will become. Another true story.

Here's something ironic in light of how comfortable I am today in my own skin. I was often ridiculed at primary school for being a bit of a weirdo. I had no boobs, a big nose, an ample bum, and a sharp mind. Clearly, the traits I carried weren't the traits that popularity demanded. But, looking back, I am super grateful that I was bullied as a child because, as an adult, it has given me a hell of a lot of resilience. Not being deemed good-looking, I compensated by developing more sustainable aspects of my personality. Funnily enough, I'm now uber-confident and capable. I now authentically own and rock my new-found sass and sense of self. Who would have thought that oddly shaped, skinny, smart kid would one day become a successful, passionate entrepreneur and fitness model?

It's time to start worrying about loving yourself instead of focusing on others loving you. When you believe in yourself, absolutely anything is possible.

4. Just be you

Embrace your individuality. The world needs you to show up for your own life and not apologise. If you try to fit in, you will never stand out. Now is the time to love your life unapologetically for yourself.

What do you see when you look in the mirror? Pain? Suffering? Fear? Beauty? Fire? Authenticity? Who would you be if you were stripped of your clothes and worldly possessions, with your soul fully exposed, baring all your truths for you to see?

In the land of social media, it's easy to fall prey to the trap of 'trying to fit in'. Behind the app-enhanced beauty and staged photographs, many social media influencers would fade into the crowd if we were to strip away the façade to expose their unaltered nakedness. News to hand… so much of what we see on social media is fake, filtered, and far from authentic and genuine.

Unfortunately, due to the veil of digital manipulation, many of these people may never experience the happiness that comes with vulnerability. True beauty comes from within. Only a naked, unashamed soul can be pure, innocent, and loved to its fullest potential.

It is an absolute certainty that no person can know their beauty or perceive a sense of their worth until it is reflected in the mirror of another loving, caring being. Love is transcendent. It knows not of time nor space and exists between us *for us*.

For me, my first husband, Brian, was an angel among us mere mortals, and he always told me that I was beautiful. At the time, and for years after he died, I never truly believed it. I have learnt from my experience as a bikini fitness comp competitor that you can have a fantastic physique, and genuine self-confidence can still shine its mighty radiance beyond the façade of the flesh. I have realised that sometimes you must be yourself and go out into the world with confidence and courage, even if you have to 'fake it till you make it'.

At heart, I'm quite a nerd. You might say I'm an 'infomaniac'. I'm the kind of person who gets cramps in their thumbs from writing fully punctuated sentences when they text. Lucky for me, I have learnt to embrace my nerdiness, but I'm also not afraid to explore other dimensions of my personality. You, too, can know how to do this.

Back in the day, I studied IT (information technology), graphic design, animation, gender studies, autobiographical writing, short film, and contemporary society at university (among many other things… I could never focus on just one subject). I now thirst for knowledge in fitness, health, and wellness. I believe in continued education, but nothing compares to life experience when you want to get something done and feel it.

Growing up, I was recognised for my intellect, not for my physical aesthetic, and, as a result, as mentioned earlier, I was teased because I was intelligent and basically 'unattractive'. I am now fundamentally grateful for this because it forced me to develop my personality, and I now possess a deep appreciation of internal radiance.

Moving into fitness modelling as a mature adult was downright frightening. It pushed my internal self way beyond the limits of my comfort zone and inherently challenged my entire perception of externality. The person I have now become is just an extension of the authentic person I have always been, only version 1.2, and, like technology, it's not backwards compatible.

The moral of the story is to let your unbridled passion for whatever you love continue to define you as a person without fear of judgement from others. The moments that define lives aren't always distinct. Be more than meets the eye.

You may not be perfect, but I'll tell you what – you can be awesome. The trick is to be yourself; I promise people will enjoy who you are. If not, forget them. Being 'you' is the most beautiful and bad-ass version of yourself that you can be. Don't worry about the haters who talk behind your back… they're behind you for a reason. I like to think that behind every bad-ass is an innocent soul who became tired of everyone's bullshit. So, I reckon you should use your haters as your motivators. The best revenge is happiness, as they say.

Sometimes we spend way too much time critiquing ourselves from the outside in. We continuously focus on those external bits of flesh, hair, teeth, or blemishes and other perceived imperfections. I see this exact behaviour play out every single day at the gym. The externality of our physical bodies is our projection of how we want people to perceive our personalities. Indeed, when did you last take the time to look yourself directly in the eyes and stare intensely at the person you are inside? How different our lives would be if only our eyes saw souls, not bodies.

It's time to love yourself, not your skin, organs, or bones, but your naked soul. Remember, our inner beauty never needs make-up or photoshop.

Don't get me wrong – I am guilty of checking myself out in the mirror in a typically shallow way. I'm human. I do feel, however, that my current external self is very much an accurate projection of the soul who now lies within… experimental, confident, vulnerable, brave, driven, and wild! Can you see the diamond that shines out to the world from behind those magnificent eyes when you catch a glimpse of yourself in the mirror? Do you recognise your authenticity? Do you abide by it, and do you trust it?

Owning our story and loving ourselves through our journey is the bravest thing we can ever do. (Side note: if you haven't read or listened to the great Brené Brown, you should). Let yourself be flawed – it makes for a much more exciting story. I have these incredible moments when I am actually in awe of my body. I have cellulite, stretch marks, asymmetry, and scars, but these are all just reminders of how much my flesh has changed and morphed into the fit body I live in today.

I challenge you to take a moment today to look yourself in the eyes in a mirror. Keeping eye contact, tell the person staring back at you – yourself – that you are perfect, wholesome, complete, loved, and enough. To borrow from Abhijit Naskar, out loud, say to yourself: "I am perfect the way I am. I am beautiful the way I am. Those who do not accept me the way I am do not deserve me in their lives."

This, of course, doesn't mean that you should never seek change and growth. It's about how and why you seek this change.

5. Momentum is the secret key to change

Yes, Momentum keeps you moving in a single direction, but it may or may not be the direction you want to head in. If you run in a downward spiral, the momentum energy will keep you down unless you take action to reverse the direction. This misguided momentum often happens when you allow your fears instead of your goals to motivate you, which is inherently counterproductive… aka… not cool!

Sometimes the only difference between kicking arse in life and getting your arse kicked by life is a few positive thoughts followed by a few positive words, all perfectly aimed in a beautifully positive direction. It's all about having your ducks in a row (as opposed to having ducks that think they're constantly at a rave!). If you do the absolute best you possibly can and come from a place of integrity, you should be proud of yourself. You don't need to give a f*ck about what anyone else thinks. If people aren't in the arena with you getting their arse kicked, don't be interested in their advice on fighting. When you feel like giving up, remind yourself that winners focus on winning, and losers focus on winners. Simple!

The truth is, the world needs me to show up for my own life – this also applies to you. We become so afraid of shining brightly because we think people will be bothered by the glare, but now that just makes me want to shine even more brightly. Better cover those eyes!

Have the courage to stand firm and tall, be yourself, and shine brightly. You won't disturb others; you'll inspire them to do the same, and you may even light someone else's candle.

A reminder that dimming someone else's light does not make yours shine more brightly. Nope. Some people play the victim to circumstances they create. You know the ones. Like me, I'm sure you have had a few 'victims' in your life who have tried to put you down.

In a way, I am grateful for their ignorance because it's now part of what made me the successful person I was always destined to become. If I were afraid, I couldn't do what I do. Sometimes you have to throw on a crown (or a cape) and remind others who they're dealing with!

Let's talk a bit about fear. Because, yes, I feel it too. I'm not immune. But with fear, we can learn to recognise that it's a positive feeling and lean into it.

I believe you have to appreciate where you've come from to know who you are and the person you would like to be.

Blessed are those whose hearts fill with the warmth of love from another. And the more love you give out, the more you get back. Energy attracts energy. Like attracts like.

DON'T LET ANYTHING KILL YOUR MOMENTUM

Before we start to gain some serious momentum, we must be aware of potential momentum killers. Every path has its pitfalls, and this

You don't need to give a f*ck about what anyone else thinks.

If people aren't in the arena with you getting their arse kicked, don't be interested in their advice on fighting.

When you feel like giving up, remind yourself that winners focus on winning, and losers focus on winners. Simple!

one is no different. You're going to meet resistance along the way, and knowing how to identify and deal with problems as they arise is key to both gaining momentum and maintaining what you have already built.

The following insights will help you keep moving forward even when times get tough.

1. Momentum has enemies

Complacency is the number one enemy of momentum. Moving forward, making progress, and achieving goals requires hard f*cking work. Identifying pain points, setting goals, making detailed plans, and taking action require effort. This is why settling and staying comfortable can appear much more natural. Nothing is worse than dwelling on the things you should do, so maybe it's time you stopped 'shoulding' all over yourself, yeah?

Culture is enemy number two. Your neighbours and co-workers may say they want to see you succeed and achieve, but they may not mean it! Brutal, right? It is a harsh reality, but it is often more convenient for someone to hold you down than to help you up – this is especially true in the workplace. So, stop worrying about other people's opinions; let them bask in their complacency and jealousy as you succeed. Boom!

2. Momentum needs maintenance

Momentum can mean the difference between a f*cking spectacular life and a mediocre one. It provides the jet fuel needed to reach your goals.

If we don't take steps to maintain it, we can lose momentum during challenging times. In our moments of suffering, it's hard to remember that the world doesn't just stop. During difficult situations, it's okay to cry, scream, shout, swear, or even be silent – whatever you need. It's okay to feel a sense of uncertainty. If everything in life were sure and defined all the time, it'd be pretty bloody dull and miserable, right? You can't feel the highs without also experiencing the lows.

Since losing Brian, I have laughed, cried, and sat in complete, perfect silence… over and over again. Honestly, it's been my life's most challenging yet cathartic period. I've serendipitously met so many incredible souls and shared their profound connective energy to such a degree that I know we are all vibing at the same level. Shout out to my tribe – you know who you are.

Let your emotional pathway of suffering be your journey to becoming unshakably unstoppable… aka getting the f*ck unstuck! Turn your most significant adversities into your ultimate advantages. You are stronger than you think.

Momentum is all about intention, habit, and balance. Here are a few practices I like to employ to ensure that I maintain momentum:

* **Be a go-getter** because conditioned, consistent activity will kick in when you finally push past an obstacle and find the time and energy you need to keep going. Too many people feel like mastery is a place you arrive at, which makes the path (momentum) vague. Mastery is a journey, and most people need to realise they still have further to go in their quest to discover their true potential. Sounds deep, I know. Bottom line – get out there and do stuff… the rest will follow.

* **Create clarity** in your life so you can see your goals. What does your ideal lifestyle look like? What are your income

goals? Focus on knowing where you are going and working out how to measure your progress. You have clear places where you want to live and visit, so be clear with your vision and purpose.

* **Avoid negativity,** and don't let people steal your dreams. One small, discouraging word from someone can stop your momentum. People will be judgemental and try to take your goals and your energy. Don't let them get you down or distract you.

* **Put out good energy and lead by example.** People will know that your intentions are good and you are doing the right thing. Believe in what you are doing. Put the good energy out there, and it will return to you in spades. I see this happen every day.

I like to balance negativity and build positive energy by using essential oils. When inhaled or applied topically, essential oils can influence areas of your brain that control stress. Essential oils can shift your mood at the physiological level, leaving you feeling more focused, energised, and prepared to take on the day and continue moving forward. And they smell bloody good!

I cannot unlearn the truths I have uncovered. I feel that I've connected with specific individuals *entirely on purpose* to discover the greater good of our mutual trajectories.

Looking back, I can see how much I've gained by focusing on momentum. The past few years have taught me a lot about the person I was, the person I am, and the person I will continue to evolve into as I continuously renew my momentum. When was the last time you laughed so hard you couldn't breathe? When did you discover a perfect moment of connection with another human being, so much so that you could cry in awe of its beauty? This is where the magic lies!

Remember, we all have the power to live with authentic joy in every moment.

Loz Lesson

To help you maintain momentum, download and complete **Daily Routine** and start mapping and prioritising your morning and evening activities to improve your daily energy and sleep quality.

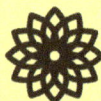

DAILY ROUTINE
TO MAINTAIN YOUR MOMENTUM

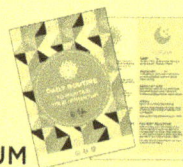

DOWNLOAD YOUR DAILY ROUTINE **lozlife.com/book-routine**

THE TRUTH ABOUT MOTIVATION

How do you feel when you open your eyes every day? Are you excited about what's to come? Or do you lack energy and motivation? The first step towards getting somewhere is to decide that you will not stay where you are, so, to help with motivation, you should set a goal that makes you want to jump out of bed in the morning.

The colder months can be demotivating because I love snuggling up in my warm bed. Because I'm not a natural morning person, it has always been a goal of mine to wake up earlier. Although I don't do it every single day, when I do make that small change, I certainly feel better about it. I have created a habit of waking up to catch the beautiful morning sun – it's always at its most stunning just after sunrise. This tiny alteration to my morning routine motivates me to walk, meditate, or do other critical, goal-related activities before I start my day. It's surprising how a small change like this gives me much more energy. It makes me want to seize the day.

Newsflash – if you want to get the f*ck unstuck, you have to think differently and choose change. Delicious, proactive, positive change. If you decide not to change, you'll end up just staying in the same place, dreaming of things you believe are out of reach.

Sometimes minor changes can make the most significant difference, so focus on your goal and remember your *motivation* and *why*. The only thing that has to stay where it's planted is a tree. Funny that.

1. The joy of missing out (JOMO)

You likely know FOMO (fear of missing out) and its cousin FOBO (fear of better options), but the next generation of tailored-for-social-media acronyms is 'JOMO', or joy of missing out. And I am here for it!

As the antithesis of FOMO, it symbolises relief from the breathless and guilt-laden need to be perennially switched on and constantly productive, which emerged in reaction to 'hustle culture' and other widely accepted models of 'success'.

At its core, JOMO means proudly living life in the slow lane and deriving pleasure from social exclusion. By intentionally taking a step back, shunning needless overexertion, and unshackling ourselves from what we 'should' be doing, fear is traded for joy. We also reclaim our most precious resource: time.

Why don't you try a little JOMO on for size?

2. Nothing happens by accident

I am in absolute awe of the energies I now attract, and I feel overwhelmingly blessed to call so many extraordinary bloody human beings "my tribe." You know who you are (and there are a lot of you!).

The universe has an incredible way of counterbalancing energy. Whenever you are down, be assured that it's not permanent because something amazingly uplifting is always around the corner if you look for it. Likewise, if you're riding on a high, in a state of ego, you can guarantee the universe will throw something at you to bring you back down. Thump. Yep. We have all been there. And it can hurt.

It's all about maintaining a universal equilibrium. Once you surrender to a power more significant than you, you will realise that no person or event *ever* manifests in your life by accident, and everything happens for a reason. Clichéd but true.

Our most prominent critics are our most outstanding teachers. Our most challenging times pose our most meaningful accomplishments. This mind-blowing realisation completely shifted my perception of time, space, and destiny. In the wise words of Dr John Demartini, one of my favourite humans, "Once you see things 'on the way' instead of 'in the way', you're set free of the bondage and burden of incomplete and one-sided emotional perspectives."[1]

At the end of it all, the greatest gift we have is our potential. Can you think of anything more horrifying than taking your last breath in this life with that potential still locked away inside you because you were too scared of not living up to the expectations of others? That won't be me! And it doesn't have to be you either. It's up to you to decide how, when, and why you will go get your dream life.

Loz Lesson

As this chapter closes, download and complete **Gratitude Tool**. This work sheet will help you anchor your intentions and find the momentum behind your *why* before we move on to the next part of the Healthy Habit Hierarchy: Menu.

GRATITUDE TOOL
5 THINGS EXERCISE

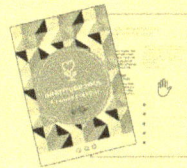

DOWNLOAD YOUR GRATITUDE TOOL **lozlife.com/book-gratitude**

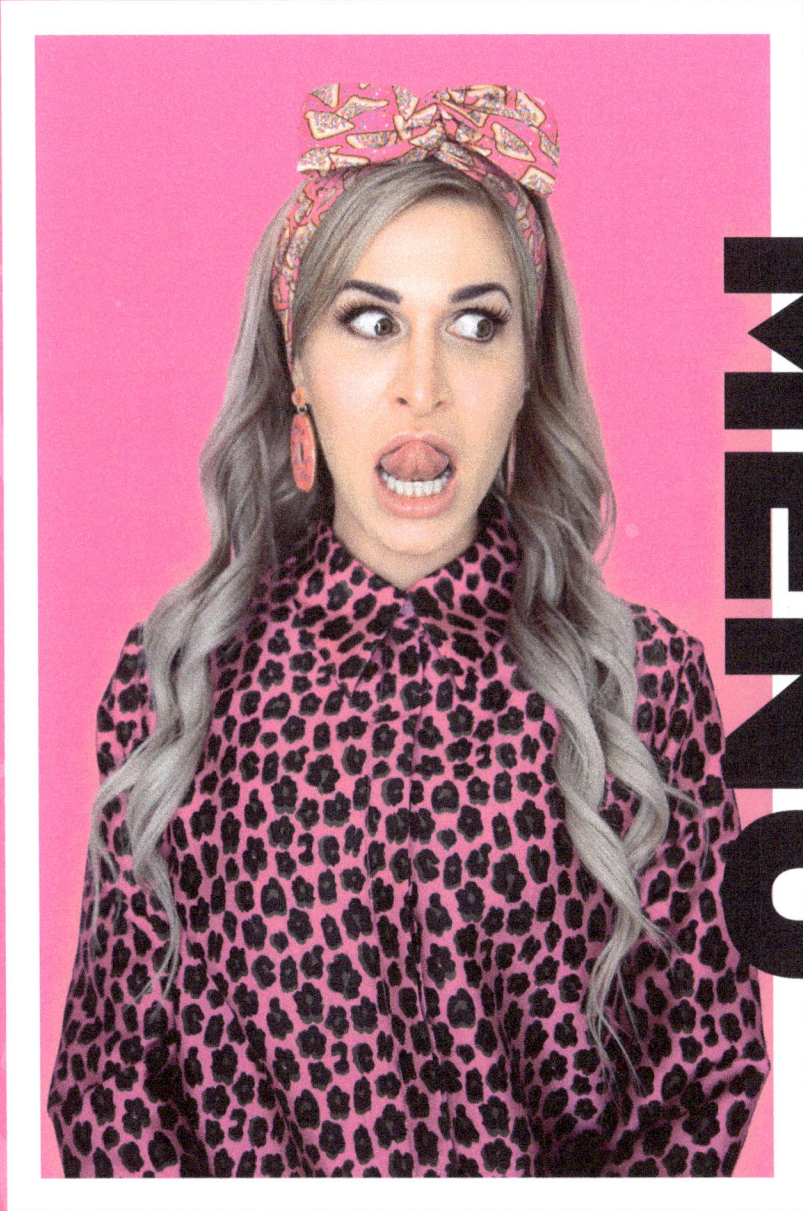

MENU

Food. Yum, right? I love to eat! And I eat a lot. I was born with food in or around my mouth. No shame.

How often have you indulged in eating something you know you shouldn't and immediately beat yourself up out of guilt? I've done it!

Your weight and how healthy you are depend a lot on your diet. Ultimately, it's the daily lifestyle choices you make, your strategy (or lack thereof), and accountability that are responsible for the habits that are destroying (or adequately fuelling) your body.

Our inherent need for fuel is at the core of optimum living and sustainable wellness. It's the force that drives us to transform the quality of our lifestyle, giving us a sense of achievement, love, and fulfilment. This energy propels us to nourish our bodies, improve our mindset, train ourselves, and boost our wealth.

Looking good and feeling great go hand in hand. Nothing tastes as good as healthy feels. If you have a healthy lifestyle, are accountable for what you put in your mouth, and move your body, you will feel freaking awesome. I believe, after you've established your *why*, optimal health 100 percent starts with food. Without quality nutritional intake, you cannot create a positive mindset, and you can't go after that positive change you seek. This is because your gut health can significantly affect your brain function.

Consequently, by addressing your food and gut health, exercise will be manageable. If you are not fuelling your mind and body to perform to your highest potential, how on earth are you supposed to maintain momentum on your path to mastery?

DO YOU FEEL TIRED A LOT OF THE TIME?

Yawn. Do you feel as though you never have any energy? Does it feel like you are always run-down, and you seem to get sick with every little bug that comes along? Do you have problems with digestion, or is it difficult to lose weight? Does your hair look flat and lifeless, and is your skin lacklustre?

If you're getting enough sleep, these signs may suggest your body is weighed down by heavy metals, chemicals, and other toxins or that your nutritional intake is not optimal. As well as being inconvenient, these factors can affect your health and how you feel daily. Who wants to feel blah? Not me.

What's your posture like over a day? Is it tall and neutral, allowing your diaphragm and nose to work effectively for good, deep, nourishing breathing patterns, or is it slumped and stooped, causing dysfunction in your uptake of air through your mouth?

It might not sound like much, but all of these symptoms matter and provide solid feedback that your body might not be running as effectively as you'd like.

THE ACCOUNTABILITY FACTOR

I am a firm believer that we can't unlock our true potential until we address what it is that we consume. A lack of accountability leads to a burden on our bodily systems. Most people ingest so much crap they cannot biochemically implement a great mindset or optimally and sustainably move their bodies. Makes sense that we sometimes feel heavy.

Do you know the seven components of food? How can you combine fats, carbohydrates, proteins, and other elements like fibre to achieve maximum health benefits? What does it mean to be and to feel nourished? Are you breathing effectively to give your brain and body the best chance to uptake oxygen?

Even though we consciously decide to eat and drink, many of us don't consider what we put into our bodies. Now is an excellent time to put down that chocolate biscuit and take a deep breath for a minute.

To strive for optimal nutrition, we must first understand the basics of food and why we should choose certain items over others. Imagine feeling content, nourished, and energised because you know how, when, and what to eat every day for the rest of your life? It's life-changing.

This chapter will help educate you about how to make better decisions regarding the types of food and beverage choices you make and how you breathe to nourish and sustain your body. By understanding your *menu*, you will be more equipped to uncover the habits holding you back from maximising your energy potential. And... yes... you'll be one step closer to being 'unstuck'.

In my experience, being overweight is just a symptom of something more profound. Interestingly, however, the

> *Fact*
>
> **You need to understand the patterns of behaviour that led you to put on the weight first *and* undertake an audit of your daily dietary consumption to avoid this weight loss being entirely unsustainable. Otherwise, you won't keep it up – or off.**

number one reason why people embark on an exercise program, join a gym, or hire a personal trainer is to lose weight. It's a bit backward if you ask me.

You must assess and modify what you are fuelling your body with to avoid putting the kilos back on or triggering a future health condition. How many people do you know who have pounded the pavement or sweated their bodies down over a '12-week challenge' only to find they end up gaining all that weight back and then some? I know a few.

As you can see, a gap exists between traditional weight loss methods (don't even start me on the fads!) and fitness protocols.

Mindset coaching and fitness programming are integral to long-term lifestyle change and the journey to fulfilment and feeling freaking awesome. Once you realise that exercising your butt off is a short-term measure, weight loss will become a by-product of mental, physical, and spiritual change. This lively meeting place will help create harmony in your life. And who doesn't want a hefty, fat, delicious dose of balance?

For me, changing what I ate and understanding my tolerance to carbohydrates had the most significant effect on my health outcomes. Yep, I used the 'C' word!

I tried a stack of diets that continually failed because I was following fads with labels attached to them – keto, Atkins, low-fat, and gluten-free, to name a few. Too often, people are confused by conflicting information and quick-fix strategies. I know I was. Sound familiar?

Trendy diets and workouts aren't the answer because those things are not sustainable. Frankly, they're a waste of time and energy.

FOOD IS YOUR PARTNER

I'm not down on dieting, but I am up on nourishing. Every time you eat, you provide yourself with the opportunity to fuel your mind and body with clean and wholesome food. Yum! Proper nutrition is essential for thinking and performing at our best. If you appreciate its natural taste, simple food nourishes your mind, body, and soul and is much better for you than medicine.

Now, I hate spending time cooking, time that I could be devoting to doing something more directly related to achieving my goals. For this reason, I plan and prepare a lot of my food in advance. That way, I minimise the time I spend thinking about what to eat and maximise the quality of what I consume. Meal prepping has changed my life!

I'm a firm believer that correct nutrition precedes any commitment to exercise. Your choice of fuel will always dictate how well your body performs. A diverse diet of clean food is fundamental to performance. Don't just chase rainbows… eat them!

To break our food down into essential components, we need to look at it in terms of the following seven elements:

1. **Carbohydrates** – You need these for energy and organ function.

2. **Fats** – Concentrated sources of energy that also make food taste better.

3. **Proteins** – Vital for energy, growth, immune function, hormones, and enzyme production.

4. **Fibre** – A mix of carbs that aren't digested. Fibre makes foods bulkier, prevents constipation, and slows nutrient absorption by causing nutrients to enter the bloodstream over a more extended period.

5. **Water** – Most of your body contains water, so it's essential for life.

6. **Vitamins** – Can be found in small quantities in food and are necessary for normal bodily function.

7. **Minerals** – also found in food and required by the body for soft tissue, skeletal, and fluid function.

Energy may not be the only basis of existence, but it is the fuel that makes everything in our lives real and possible. Educating yourself and making small changes to your routine today will point you towards achieving your goals, maintaining a healthy lifestyle, and reducing your body fat percentage. Win-win-win!

USING YOUR MENU TO MAXIMISE YOUR MINDSET AND MOVEMENT

Food – we either love it, hate it, or don't know what to do with it.

Unfortunately, we can't just take some magic pill to make our bodies perform at their best. Yes, supplements exist, but they're just that: supplements. Their real purpose is to supplement the fuel (food) we put into our biological machine (our bodies) to perform optimally, not to replace it.

Creating healthy consumption habits comes down to education and accountability. How often have you been guilty of mindless munching because you were bored? If prompted, could you recall all the food and beverages you consumed over the past 24 hours?

Did you know that the daily choices we make have a profound effect on our cellular health? This means that the way we treat our body has a more significant impact than the genetics we inherited from our parents. The good news is that you are in control.

The decisions we make, directly and indirectly, profoundly affect our DNA. Some of us take supplements and exercise, and some of us don't. The question is, are we biohacking our bodies or hijacking our health?

When it comes to health, the most common mistake people make is only focusing on weight loss, or how much they weigh. That's why fat burners exist and why liposuction and diet fads have skyrocketed in popularity. We all want a quick fix. As world-leading life strategist and health advocate, Tony Robbins, says, "Who cares if you're putting endless amounts of cholesterol and saturated fats into your body – you look great."[2]

Most people fail at keeping the weight off by returning to regular habits. Nothing like a good yo-yo diet. They have nothing left to show for the torture they put their body through, and they may have even created irreparable damage to their health and wellness.

So, do you go ketogenic? Paleo? Plant-based? How do you find a diet that won't just help you shed that weight but will improve your overall health? Do you try some crazy breathwork fad and have ice baths? How do you find the path that will lead to lasting change? Big questions!

To make better choices about our menu, we must first identify what we are currently consuming and how we breathe. When did you last check the food pyramid? We have been conditioned to believe that cereal, milk, and cured meats are the right paths to nutrition. However, eating half a loaf of white bread a day doesn't get you the body you want. It may give you speedy energy, but most bread products contain preservatives and additives like food dyes or high fructose corn syrup – does not sound delicious.

THE NEW FOOD PYRAMID

Dr Steven Gundry is a renowned functional medicine specialist who has revolutionised the traditional food pyramid. His ideology for healthy eating aligns your food choices with the approach of modern functional medicine, looking at the body as one integrated system in which everything connects. Functional medicine seeks to identify and address the root causes of health problems rather than treating symptoms in isolation. So, for example, weight gain (or loss) is not treated separately but as a symptom of underlying health or behavioural problems. Makes so much sense.

Inspired by the Gundry Food Strategy, I have created my own eating framework by combining it with the philosophy of Simon Hill from The Proof, a plant-based-living movement.[3] The overall objective of the New Food Pyramid is to improve health, happiness, and longevity by making simple changes to the diet. The best part of this approach to food? You can efficiently address common health problems by identifying patterns and interrupting habits that might not necessarily be conducive to long-term vitality.

The earlier you tackle your wellness goals and start working on your menu, the sooner you can make your menu an essential part of your life. If you are habitually doing it, you won't have to think about it.

The first step to reaching your goal is to clearly understand where you are right now, where you want to be, and how to get there. You may have a plan for your business, career, and even your relationship… why not your health?

Considering the bigger picture, you can narrow it down to what habits need building and what healthier practices could and should replace the not-so-healthy ones.

THE NEW FOOD PYRAMID

Inspired by
DR GUNDRY &
PLANT PROOF

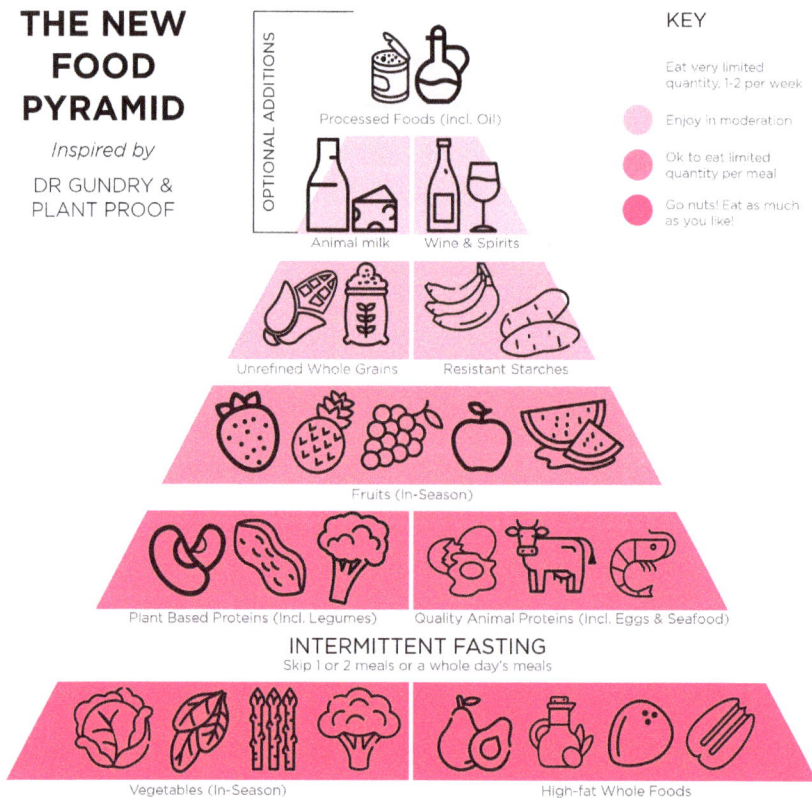

OPTIONAL ADDITIONS

Processed Foods (incl. Oil)

Animal milk   Wine & Spirits

Unrefined Whole Grains   Resistant Starches

Fruits (In-Season)

Plant Based Proteins (incl. Legumes)   Quality Animal Proteins (incl. Eggs & Seafood)

INTERMITTENT FASTING
Skip 1 or 2 meals or a whole day's meals

Vegetables (In-Season)   High-fat Whole Foods

KEY

Eat very limited quantity, 1-2 per week

Enjoy in moderation

Ok to eat limited quantity per meal

Go nuts! Eat as much as you like!

FOODS TO LIMIT
- Refined Starchy Foods: Rice, bread, cereal, pastry, potatoes, flour & cookies
- Pumpkin seeds, sunflower seeds, peanuts & cashews
- Sunflower & canola oils

FOODS TO RECONSIDER
- Sugar, aspartame & most artificial sweeteners
- Soy, grape-seed, corn, peanut & cottonseed oils

Loz Lesson

To kickstart your Menu journey, download and complete **Meal Planner** to start thinking about the delicious meals you can create using The New Food Pyramid.

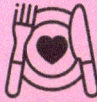

MEAL PLANNER

FOOD PYRAMID

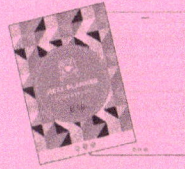

DOWNLOAD YOUR MEAL PLANNER **lozlife.com/book-meal**

CLIENT STORY
– REWRITING THE MENU

Helping clients get their menus in order isn't always just about laying out a healthy eating blueprint. Sometimes, before we can take action, we must identify what is causing someone to adopt and maintain unhealthy habits in the first place.

Courtney had hit a very low point in her life. She was once a national level athlete but after a destructive break-up from a long-term relationship, she had found herself turning to food to cope with her emotions. Consequently, Courtney gained 40 kg in a short time and was struggling to even get motivated to get out of bed and go to work at a large supermarket. Her lethargy was through the roof, and so was her blood pressure. She had developed reflux, bloating, and headaches. She spoke with her GP, who suggested she join a gym to manage her weight and consider bariatric surgery. Courtney joined a local gym, and I met her when she did one of my Pilates classes on a Tuesday evening.

We chatted briefly after class, and Courtney decided to book a discovery call with me, thinking the outcome would be that she would hire me as a personal trainer to help her get fit. This, however, would not be the case.

When we broke down where she was in her life, where she wanted to be, and why she wasn't there yet, Courtney realised that she had not taken the time to deal with her emotions since her break-up. She had cut herself off from her support network and just stopped giving a shit about what she shoved in her mouth. She felt unworthy of love and was self-sabotaging her future happiness to sit in a victim mentality because receiving people's sympathy was kinda making her feel valued. When we hit this deep spot, she cried so much, but something shifted inside her when she realised what she was doing.

Rather than unpacking all the emotional baggage she was dragging behind her, we focused on Courtney's eating. With a clear framework and measurable milestones, I knew that the skills she had developed as an athlete would be completely transferable when it came to discipline and accountability. By focusing *just* on eating, I guaranteed Courtney that she would notice symptom improvement and, eventually, find more mental bandwidth to tackle the turmoil of her break-up. We also chatted about how it was impossible to out-exercise a suboptimal diet.

For the next 12 weeks, Courtney undertook my Weight Loz program, where we checked in weekly. I provided her with a simple eating blueprint to help her gain control of her habits, and we tracked her progress, celebrating all the small wins along the way. With this plan, Courtney not only completely eradicated all her digestive symptoms, but her energy skyrocketed; her weight went back down to what it had been before shit hit the fan, and she finally found the confidence to date again, in her early 40s.

SIMPLE STEPS FOR SIGNIFICANT CHANGES

When it comes to enhancing your menu, there are some essential things you need to keep in mind. You're building a lifestyle that will get you to your ultimate goal, so these healthy habits will keep you on your journey towards mastery. Simple is always best.

1. Undertake a Metabolic Reboot

As part of my Healthy Habit Hierarchy, a reboot is the first phase of my clients' commitment to change. For many people embarking on a journey to lifelong wellness, it is by far the most challenging yet most important and rewarding step. This short phase ensures that your system is rebooted and that you're creating a level playing field. It's about getting the foundation right. You can then make long-term improvements to your mindset and movement.

Essentially a detox, the primary goal behind a reboot is to bring your body back to a baseline using a simplified, low-inflammatory diet rich in nutrients. This process helps us purge substances from the body that might be increasing the toxic load on our system and also helps to address our carbohydrate intake. There's that 'C' word again. It's not all bad; I promise.

Because the reboot phase varies from person to person, it can go from five to ten days, based upon various factors unique to each person's situation. A reboot aims to give our organs a rest, help flush toxins, and detoxify our whole internal system. Metabolic capacity increases through the process, and the basal metabolic rate significantly lifts, provided you stick to your reboot 100 percent. Increasing your metabolism is a good thing.

While many types of cleanses exist today, detoxes are becoming quite popular. Herbal detoxes have gained momentum as a simple tool for weight loss. Detoxification was previously associated with treatments to assist with dependence upon drugs and alcohol. Today, the term 'detox' is associated with herbs and particular diets that can help eliminate harmful substances from the body for overall general health.

The process of detoxification itself is a natural process for removing toxins from your body. Toxins are anything that could hurt the body. During the reboot, toxins transform into compounds, such as urine or stools, and are then excreted from the body.

Several sources of toxins may be detrimental to your overall vitality. Sometimes, the body itself can produce toxins through perfectly normal bodily functions. An excellent example of this is the production of ammonia when protein is broken down by the body. Other possible toxins include:

* Drugs
* Pesticides
* Air pollution
* Cigarette smoke
* Food additives
* Heavy metals
* Household cleaners

Benefits of a Reboot

A reboot can be beneficial for many reasons, as it cleanses the body of chemicals. Researchers believe that we consume a plethora of chemicals daily through our air, water, and food.[4] It's thought that these chemicals become deposited within our fat cells, leading to long-term health problems. Although it's nice to believe that the body will cleanse itself of these toxins, if dietary choices lack nutrients, the body's natural ability to detoxify itself is diminished. Oxidative stress can subsequently accumulate in the body through the continuous build-up of toxins. Over time, this may amount to levels that can potentially interfere with our body's capacity to function optimally and may contribute to the development of a range of chronic health conditions.[5] Yes, people, toxins are nasty!

For me, the burden of caffeine and oxidative stress tended to overload my body, especially when preparing for a bikini fitness competition. This massive load is known as a 'body burden', and researchers think it could result in many health problems, such as impaired immune function, hormonal imbalances, nutritional deficiencies, and a dysfunctional metabolism.[6]

Symptoms of these health problems can include:

* Indigestion   * Muscle pain

* Fatigue   * Bad breath

* Dull skin or breakouts

There are undoubtedly many benefits to a reboot protocol, and increased energy is a primary benefit. Even those who exercise regularly may experience a lack of energy at some point in life, feeling drained and not understanding why. Among other factors, a build-up of toxins inside the body could be the reason, and a reboot may relieve these symptoms and reboot the system. See ya later, toxins.

Additionally, a reboot may provide other benefits for the general population. A reboot may help you feel healthier throughout the year if you are prone to frequent illnesses. Notably, during cold and flu season, you may find that your natural processes slow down, making it difficult for your body to fight off viruses. Further, toxins slow down your immune system during this time, making it easier to become ill.

Rebooting can make it easier for the body to digest food, which can help relieve symptoms, such as indigestion, and decrease stomach pain and headaches.

Another benefit may be improved mental clarity by clearing 'brain fog', as toxins in our body may slow down cognition. When your body is clean of toxins, it can be easier to think more clearly and deal with day-to-day challenges.

A reboot basically consists of the following steps:

* **Include high-quality foods** (preferably organic) that provide the vital nutrients, vitamins, and antioxidants the body requires for detoxification.

* **Consume adequate water and high-fibre foods** that work to draw out and then eliminate toxins from the body.

* **Add a polyphenol-rich supplement into your diet** to
  help improve the ratios of your healthy gut bacteria and
  rid your body of the types of bacteria that feed on sugars.
  Polyphenols are organic compounds found in the seeds,
  skins, and peels of foods that help us maintain balance in
  our gut. Unfortunately, we tend to undereat them in our
  standard Western diet.

* **Retrain yourself to breathe through your nose**
  instead of your mouth. Functional breathing is so
  powerful. Life-changing, even. Most people suffer from
  dysfunctional and shallow breathing. Correct oral posture
  and an optimised breathing technique are essential for
  digestion and vitality. Since the introduction of sugar to
  our diets, many of us now mouth breathe due to nasal
  congestion caused by high sugar intake, and our tongues
  do not sit snug at the roof of our mouths when we are
  resting.[7] This can impact our airways and impede our
  capacity to breathe adequate oxygen. It's well documented
  that mouth-breathing adults are more likely to experience
  lower sleep quality, decreased productivity, and poorer
  quality of life than those who nasal breathe.[8] Get nose
  breathing, people.

* **Focusing on eliminating caffeine, alcohol, tobacco, and
  sugar** (CATS). We all know that too much of any of these
  things has a massive impact on long-term health outcomes.
  Consider swapping out coffee for invigorating herbal teas,

alcohol for sparkling water, tobacco for some time in nature, and sugar for exercise. It sounds crazy, but these alternatives can stimulate oxytocin (your 'love hormone') to make you feel good.

Consult your trusted health care provider before undertaking a reboot to ensure you do not compromise your long-term health, especially if you have diabetes.

Reboot Basics

* **Start each day of your reboot by drinking at least a half to 1 litre of water with some freshly squeezed lemon juice,** ideally one hour before your first meal. This will help you with digestion, stimulate your vagus nerve, and activate bodily functions.

* **Follow the Specific Carbohydrate Diet,** which contains no starchy carbohydrates.[9] Don't cheat! If you aren't supposed to have something, don't.

* **Drink lots of water.** Water will help with the reboot process and will also help to curb your hunger if needed – so you must consume 2 to 4 litres per day.

* **Sugar is not allowed.** Yes, this can be a challenge if you have a sweet tooth, but eliminating sugar will help reduce inflammation and will starve your harmful bacteria.

* **No pre-mixed alcohol,** as most of these beverages are just sugar and carbohydrates, so this is a big no-no!

* **Sleep a lot,** as you only recover while you're sleeping. Sleep will also help to reset your body clock and help your body burn fat. Clearing your schedule may help maximise reboot results.

* **Ensure you have salt.** A pinch or two of pink Himalayan rock salt on your meal is ideal.

* **Do things that make you feel good.** Engage in activities that train your mind to be willing to search for positivity. Self-care is essential, so take time to look after yourself during the process. Why not book a massage, learn to meditate, go for a long walk, or treat yourself to something that makes you feel good on your terms?

* **Use a daily supplement** containing an abundance of polyphenols to help control the growth of gut bacteria by killing the bad stuff and helping you thrive.

A reboot will help create a more effective process whereby your body can burn fat stores as fuel during the detox. Your body will come out of the reboot in a heightened state – it will be more sensitive to the stimulus you then expose it to (that is, food and exercise), which is precisely the outcome you want. Once you have completed the reboot, the trick is to slowly introduce carbs into your diet. A reboot will recalibrate your metabolism to use your menu more effectively, meaning fuel will burn more intensely.

Because of this, you will experience a boost in your insulin sensitivity, which is essential when higher loads of carbohydrates are introduced back into your regular menu. The reboot will kickstart your digestive tract, preparing it to utilise the high doses of nutrients consumed after the reset phase.

Your body will be more likely to use sugar effectively and maintain stable blood sugar levels. Accordingly, you will avoid insulin resistance, one of the main symptoms of diabetes. As a plus, your body will be able to handle protein more effectively, helping you build more lean muscle when you reach the movement phase of the Healthy Habit Hierarchy.

During the reboot process, be prepared to endure a few bouts of low energy, headaches, fatigue, and frustration, but know that you're doing great for your metabolism. Chances are, before this reboot, you won't have put much consideration into the breakdown of what you've been consuming in terms of proteins, fats, and carbohydrates. You perhaps also would not have given much thought to the importance of the timing of your meals, the types of carbohydrates or fats you've been ingesting, or the level of health in your digestive tract and gut. That changes now.

Embarking on a reboot in the early stages of your wellness journey will ensure that any exercise you undertake as you progress through the Healthy Habit Hierarchy will best benefit your body. You may even find that your palate changes and you no longer crave starchy carbs or sugary foods. Can you imagine not craving sugar every afternoon?

Even better, if you choose a calorie deficit eating regimen for weight loss after your reboot (that is, consuming less energy than you're outputting through exercise), you will change your body composition towards a healthy and sustainable physique.

Loz Lesson

Ready for a reboot? Learn more about my
10-Day Reboot to start feeling better sooner!

10 DAY REBOOT

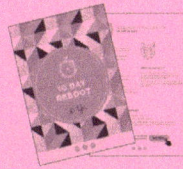

DOWNLOAD YOUR 10 DAY REBOOT **lozlife.com/book-reboot**

2. Create a Balanced Diet

A good foundation for your menu plan is figuring out how many calories you need to be consuming. The reality is that the majority of the population either undereat or overeat. Your optimum calorie intake is based on what you put into your body (input) and how much you exercise (output). At its core, it's a pretty straightforward case of mathematics. Please stick with me here. There are a lot of other essential factors to consider when we aim for lifelong balance. Macro and micronutrient breakdowns of ingredients are essential, and the amount of food we consume daily is a crucial measure of calorific significance.

To achieve your body goals, you need to establish a healthy and achievable level of water, protein, carbs, and fat consumption and stick to it. Your body needs all these things to function correctly, especially if exercise is part of your lifestyle.

There are calculators on the internet that will help you find out what your calorie intake should be. Your ideal daily consumption will be based on certain variables, such as your age, stats, and activity level.

My favourite calculator can be found on the Calorie Counter Australia website (www.caloriecounter.com.au/calorie-calculator). Just enter your age, sex, height, weight, and activity level, and it will provide you with a breakdown of daily calorie intake options based on your goals. Once you know where you sit with your daily food intake, you can easily adjust your diet to match your exercise level as you introduce movement into your lifestyle during your ascent through the Healthy Habit Hierarchy. You can then create a trackable and sustainable system to help you achieve your goals in no time.

There are several great smartphone apps, such as MyFitnessPal, or you could create a food journal to record all the food and drinks you consume over a day. It's also helpful to note how you were feeling before and during eating. These tools can help you stay accountable to your goals and see if you have unhealthy eating patterns that may be triggered by thoughts, emotions, or responses to specific events.

Loz Lesson

Once you have established your target
daily calorie intake, download and complete
Shopping List to simplify your food shopping.
And don't forget to plan for a weekly
meal prep session.

SHOPPING LIST
FOOD PYRAMID

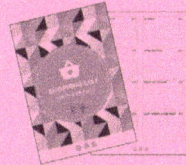

DOWNLOAD YOUR SHOPPING LIST **lozlife.com/book-shopping**

3. Get to Know Your Metabolism

The next step is understanding your metabolism. How many people do you know who can eat everything they want and still stay skinny? You might be one of them, but the truth is it's pretty tough for such people to gain weight and muscle (and some of them want to). Ironically, many people want to lose weight, while many would love nothing more than to gain it.

Think of your metabolism like a fire: when you add a log of quality firewood (that is, wholesome foods, such as high-quality protein, slow-burning low-GI carbohydrates, and healthy fats), the fire burns longer. When you don't put a log on the fire or when you add wet tinder (like refined carbohydrates and sugary foods), the fire dies down or fizzles out.

I deal with many clients who have a low tolerance for carbohydrates. Understanding your carbohydrate tolerance is crucial for lasting health and wellness. I need a lot of carbs to get through my day, which is why carbs are not bad, and I can consume a high level of carbohydrates without gaining weight. I have a threshold, though; if I cross it regularly, I will definitely stack on the kilos.

Understanding your metabolism is essential when trying to reach your body goals, but it's not as easy as it seems. You might need help from an expert. If you struggle to lose weight, you could choose to leave your weight loss journey to trial and error. However, for more practical and long-term weight loss success, getting the right advice and having someone to keep you accountable is the safest and fastest route to creating lasting results. It's a fact!

Seeking good professional guidance can help you tailor your balanced diet to your health and medical history. These professionals can provide additional advice or recommendations to improve your health. Your doctor, aware of your health and medical conditions, can give tips about certain foods. Or they can provide advice about an eating pattern to help you achieve a balanced diet and improve your overall health. You may also receive a referral to a local dietitian.

A well-stocked pantry can be an excellent tool for maintaining a balanced diet. If you are active, like me, stock up on foods that offer a quick, easy, balanced meal.

These staples include:

* Any beans in a can

* Canned vegetables (no salt)

* Tuna

* Brown rice or 100 percent whole-wheat pasta

* Nut butter (I love almond butter)

* Frozen vegetables with no seasoning or sauces

* Frozen fruits

* Pre-cooked brown rice or quinoa

* Low-carb frozen dinners (for busy nights... but be aware of high salt)

* Frozen proteins (fish, beef, lamb, pork, chicken, or tempeh)

* A supply of fresh lean proteins (chicken, fish, pork, or lean beef) and fruits and vegetables

If you're busy with work, juggling a hundred things at once, and don't have the time to cook a delicious meal, supplements could be the best way to ensure your menu is sustainable and easy to follow, even on a busy schedule. In saying that, I certainly don't believe everyone needs them. I suggest only using them after you've been following an optimised diet for a while because some people – especially men – rely on them to see results, which is unsustainable. Nonetheless, a good quality multi-omega and non-synthetic multivitamin is definitely a combination I recommend most people take for overall vitality.

So now you know the elements of a balanced diet, let's talk about how you can turn it into a habit that will form part of your new optimised lifestyle. Yes, it's an integral part of moving from stuck to unstoppable.

4. Turn Your Diet into a Part of Your Lifestyle

My first coach told me, "If you want to change your life, start with your environment." If you're going to make your diet more sustainable, you can't do it without a bit of change.

So, if you are ready to start, clean the fridge and throw away sugars: sauces, marinades, fruit juices, and chocolate. I know, I know, it sounds painful… but I promise you'll feel super proud of yourself. Go on. I'll wait here while you do it.

The best way to stop binging on unhealthy foods is to replace them with healthy and delicious alternatives. And no, I don't just mean carrots.

Here are a few tips:

* If you crave something sweet, have a piece of low-carb fruit like rockmelon or a couple of strawberries.

* Apply the 80/20 rule, which means if you follow your diet 80 percent of the time and allow yourself an indulgence 20 percent of the time, you're doing just fine!

✱ Prepare, prepare, prepare… it is the key to success. If you have healthy food on hand and ready to go, you are less likely to reach for impulse foods like sugar-laden snacks.

You are building a lifestyle and need to make it sustainable, but, unfortunately, people end their wellness journey by forcing themselves to do something they don't want to do. To make your goals long-term, you must stick with them, even after achieving them. It would be best if you convinced yourself to continue with your healthy habits, and having a network of supportive peers – aka a tribe of like-minded souls – can make this a lot easier.

5. Create a Support Network

It can be daunting to embark on a journey to change your lifestyle if you feel like you're doing it all alone. I can certainly attest to having felt this myself. One is the loneliest number, after all. If you live and work with other people, it is essential to discuss how to manage food so they can help support your goal of creating healthier eating habits.

Having family members, friends, or workmates as food supporters will make it easier for you to make good decisions when it comes to choosing a healthy menu. And they may even be inspired to join you.

6. Start Tracking Your Sleep

Today, we're fortunate to have access to fantastic wearable technology that allows us to track sleep. There's an abundance of options at your disposal – from wristbands and smart watches to unique rings on your finger that contain sensors and microchips. No matter which option you choose, they'll typically track a stack of biometric data and, at the same time, your sleep, including your heart rate (HR), heart rate variability (HRV), respiratory rate, body temperature, and, more importantly, your stages of sleep.

Each device typically works with a separate app that gives you results on your mobile device. I prefer devices that don't have screens (like a ring) so they have zero impact on my sleep through junk blue light.

Remember, you can only improve what you can measure, so doing your homework on the best device and taking the time to understand how to interpret the information it provides will create a clear starting point for your sleep-tracking journey.

We will talk more about sleep in the next chapter – I just wanted you to start thinking about it now!

REMEMBER, IT'S ALL ABOUT HAVING A FLEXIBLE YET BALANCED DIET

A flexible diet is best if you want to stay motivated and inspire yourself towards your goal. Alternative diets (vegetarian, low-fat, keto) are defined with stringent rules and are not always compatible with your preferences or tastes. In my opinion, if your diet has an official title, you shouldn't be following it! The label generally equals a fad.

Of course, rules are essential, but a flexible diet is far from being as strict as other diets. A flexible menu opens up people's choices. It takes the pressure off. Eating various vegetables and nutritious wholefoods, such as quality meats, plant-based proteins, and good fats is encouraged, but there is no strict rule of eating only certain types of food.

Initially, creating an optimal diet is primarily about establishing a daily calorie target – the most crucial factor in weight control. Feeling bored or beholden to strict food lists and recipes can get old quickly. However, if you stick to the basic principles of consuming quality, fresh, nutritious wholefoods, with low carbohydrates and fats, you can be flexible and eat the foods you enjoy in moderation.

Remember, no one knows you better than you do. While you can get advice from a fitness or nutrition coach, you are the only person to set the goals for you. What do you want to do, and what are you willing to sacrifice? Where do you want your dreams to take you, and are you ready to start the journey?

So, the first step – decide what you are going to do. If you want a great way to benchmark your current body composition, get a body composition scan known as a DEXA (dual-energy X-ray absorptiometry). A DEXA will show you how much muscle and fat you have, including fat around your organs, and your bone density. You can access this type of scan at most major radiography centres for a fee and without a doctor's referral.

Once you have decided how and why you want to improve your eating habits, you can design your ideal menu and *plan your meals in advance whenever possible*. It's not as hard as it sounds – there are many free resources online.

Remember, documenting your progress will help you stay accountable to your plan as you continuously measure your improvement until you reach your destination. Weigh yourself once a week and take regular measurements of your waist, hips, and chest. Use a journal, take progress photos, and note any changes to the way your clothes fit and any improvements in your daily energy levels. Setting goals, motivating yourself, and making the whole experience successful and enjoyable are paramount to creating healthy eating habits. And don't forget to celebrate all the little victories along the way. But maybe not with a tub of ice cream…

As you can see, there's much more to the food you're eating than you probably realised. To quote Hippocrates, "Let food be thy medicine and medicine be thy food." It's essential to make sure you're choosing the best food to keep you happy and healthy long term, to fuel your life.

Loz Lesson

To help you plan to succeed, download **You Can Do It!** Over the next week, use this tracking tool to record everything you eat and drink. Remember, sauces, dressings, and incidental cappuccinos add up over days, weeks, and months.

YOU CAN DO IT!
KEEP TRACK

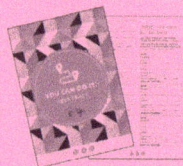

DOWNLOAD YOUR KEEP TRACK EXERCISE **lozlife.com/book-do-it**

Without knowing how much or how little fuel you consume daily, it's challenging to break the cycle of not-so-great habits. These unconscious eating, drinking, and breathing patterns can lead to long-term fatigue and general suboptimal wellness. And this is a pretty shitty place to get stuck.

If you find yourself binging on something naughty, make a note about any emotional triggers that may have led you to choose that particular food (for example, "I was upset because…" or, "I was nervous because…"). At the end of the week, look back at what you consumed and see if you can identify any eating patterns linked to specific emotional triggers. You might be surprised.

That said, don't be hard on yourself. We all do it. We all stuff up. Just get back on the horse, my friend.

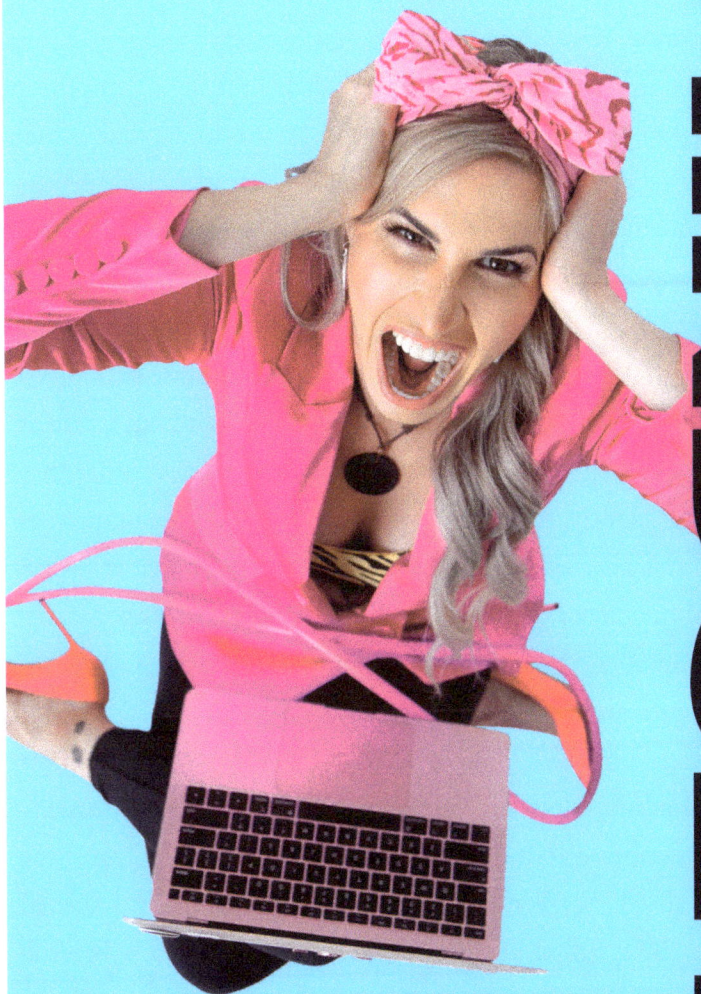

MINDSET

f we focus on the trail of stress, it will lead to our deepest fear. Tony Robbins explains, "If you're going to succeed at the highest level, you've got to face your fears."[10] But fears are, by their very definition, scary!

What are your biggest fears? Are your beliefs limiting or empowering you? Do you push through your fear or let it cripple you? When was the last time you took a moment to pause, breathe, and feel the energy you subconsciously create?

Most of us don't know how to control our thoughts, so, instead, we let them control us. Unfortunately, though, our minds will never make us happy. The truth is we need to unlock our fears because the biggest handbrakes in our life are our beliefs about ourselves and our world as a whole. The challenge with most of our current theories is that they develop subconsciously. Although this can be scary, if we can uncover those habits that restrict the unleashing of our true potential, it can also be one of the most exciting processes of our lives. So empowering!

In your moments of fear, it's impossible to love yourself. Without reasonable confidence, you cannot be successful or happy. When you believe in your capabilities, this confidence will become the most beautiful and admirable trait you can rock. This is why it's equally important to celebrate your little wins when things don't go your way.

When I realised that beneath my fear was vulnerability, I started to notice that life is full of beauty; I realised it's okay to stop, breathe, and relax. Fear exists in a moment. Go around and see the butterfly, the small child, and the smiling faces. Smell the rain and feel the wind. Live your life. Live it to its fullest potential, and fight for your big-arse dreams.

Growing up, I suffered from low self-esteem, and one of my biggest fears was not fitting in. This fear followed me into my adult life, where I would undertake many ventures for external validation. I had no clue who I was – I was living for everyone else.

Eventually, sometime around my early 30s, I reached a point where I identified how much energy living in an unauthentic state was consuming. At this very point, I started accepting myself for who I was. If you didn't take me the way I was, you weren't meant to be in my life. See ya!

I now do what I do, inspiring others, to harness pure fulfilment. I want to be a great role model for women, men, youth – all human beings. What you see is what you get with me. Proudly so.

I want to be authentic. Within my community, I want to be viewed as a natural, flawed person and not be put on a pedestal. I'm human. I make mistakes, cry, hurt, and love… just like you. Moving forward with authentic joy occurred when I realised that my ego – that part that wants to feel validated through feelings of significance – wouldn't encourage me. Ahhh, the ego. She can be quite the beast!

Deep fulfilment can be accomplished when we let go of our ego. When we match our highest values to meaningful actions, we add value to the lives of others, and this, in turn, provides a very satisfying sense of happiness. Who doesn't want to feel happy?

Have you ever noticed that everyone laughs the same all over the world? Laughter is a universal connection and if you laugh a lot, your wrinkles will always be in the right places as you age. A bit of raw happiness doesn't need botox. In my eyes, a day without laughter is a day wasted. As the saying goes, laughing may not add years to your life, but it certainly will add life to your years. You must admit, life is always better when you smile! And yes, I try to make everyone around me laugh, but sometimes they joke about me, and I'm okay with that. Learning to laugh at yourself is quite a gift!

It's time to love yourself, not your skin, organs, or bones but your naked soul.

Remember, our inner beauty never needs makeup or photoshop.

MINDFULNESS AND MEDITATION

Here's the thing I have noticed about laughter. When I laugh, I am very mindful of that moment. Mindfulness and meditation are often used interchangeably, which can be confusing. In simple terms, 'meditation' is an ancient attention-training technique, while 'mindfulness' is a practical attitude or approach for practising meditation. I believe in the power of both.

We all know that mindfulness can help us feel better, be calmer, and 'amp up' our self-care. But did you know that practising mindfulness can be a helpful tool when you want to assess how your daily activities are supporting you? It's not just about the warm and fuzzies. A mindful connection can guide you and your daily direction, so what better time to regain clarity and focus than right now?

Mindfulness is the awareness that occurs when we non-judgementally pay attention to the present moment. Equally important, meditation helps bring this awareness to a specific focal point, training your mind to focus your attention consciously.

Back in the day, meditation was reserved for your weird friend's equally odd parents. You know, the ones with the house full of crystals, bells, and exotic music. But as it turns out, they might have been onto something!

Modern scientific research into the benefits of practising meditation is increasingly revealing some fantastic things. As it turns out, meditation is a wellness powerhouse, with benefits that include reduced stress levels, increased capacity to manage pain, improved focus, better connection with others, and greater self-acceptance!

As meditation becomes more mainstream, you may wonder why you should try it. These are the science-backed benefits. Meditation can:

* Reduce stress

* Help control anxiety

* Increase mindfulness

* Encourage mental wellness and good emotional health

* Improve self-awareness

* Improve focus and attention span

* Slow age-related memory problems

* Help tackle addictions

* Improve sleep

* Help control pain

* Reduce blood pressure

* Help you feel kinder[11]

Scientific research into meditation shows that it is a potent tool for increasing your wellbeing and health, so I guess the question is... why not?

Like the art of mindfulness, meditation is where we adopt the attitude of a curious observer of our mind and our subconscious and notice what is happening without judging it as good or bad. A non-judgemental approach enables you to see more clearly what is happening rather than reacting from fear, bias, or prejudice, which often distort insight. In this particular meditative practice, we focus on our senses to create a state of calmness by aligning internal and external energies with our focus.

As you can see, both mindfulness and meditation make you more aware of what's happening in your subconscious mind by connecting to the present moment. Both help you identify your limiting beliefs and biggest fears and can tap into an unconscious sense of calm and happiness. Unlocking your deepest fears will help uncover the patterns holding you back from unleashing your true potential. This self-discovery can be one of your life's most challenging but exciting processes. And… you guessed it… can help you feel free and unstoppable.

In this chapter, you will learn that it's possible to turn crisis into opportunity and to feel authentic joy. I know because I have done and continue to do this myself. Every day.

DO YOU HAVE JUST TEN MINUTES?

We live in a busy world. The pace is often frantic, and our minds are always active. In moments of supposed relaxation, we are still often mindlessly doing something.

I'd like you to take a moment to think back to when you last took time out to do nothing. I'm talking *ten total minutes* of wholly uninterrupted time, a time when you did nothing at all. No TV, no chatting, no emailing, no reading, no SMS, no planning, just simply doing nothing. Can you even think of having had such a time? Perhaps you can't even comprehend the idea of doing nothing.

Modern life can be sad, and the extraordinary reality is that most of us don't regularly take quality time out to 'be'. Our mind is our most precious resource, and we use it to experience many moments. Our brain helps us to be content, happy, thoughtful, considerate, and kind to others. When it comes to our mind, let's face it, we don't always look after it. We take it for granted. We spend far more time thinking about our clothes, cars, and hair than we ever want to admit... Okay, maybe it's just me who obsesses over hair!

We become stressed because we don't stop and look after our minds. I liken this monkey mind to a washing machine going around and around. If your complicated emotions were coloured clothes and your confusing thoughts were your whites, you'd end up with a bit of a mess if you washed them all together. The trouble is that we mix emotions with thoughts so damn frequently, and we are conditioned so profoundly in our behavioural patterns that most don't know how to deal with it. With multiple attention-sapping distractions, we're no longer aware of the world, and we miss things that should be most important to us, like moments. Mindful moments. The crazy thing is that so many of us assume that's the way life is, so we've just got to get on with it. When there is the constant wandering of the mind, we tend to be unhappy.

Since I worked all this out, I realised how much I love being in the present moment. Sadly, most of us spend little time in the 'here and now', but I have some good news: that's not how it has to be.

I once read that if you place one foot in the future and the other in the past, you're pissing on the present. Excellent quote, right? Living in the now sounds easy, but research from Harvard suggests that our minds are lost in thought almost 47 percent of the time.[12] Yes, 47 percent! Of course, 'thinking time' is crucial to mental development. Still, it seems tragic that half of our lives are potentially lost through counterproductive, distractive thoughts instead of just being in the moment.

Luckily for you, it doesn't need to be that way. There are proven techniques that enable our minds to be less distracted and more mindful. I use these tools so frequently that I have conditioned myself to break free of obsessive anxiety. By engaging in short but frequent mindfulness practices throughout my day, I now live a life that is extraordinarily anxiety-free and happy. Yep, it's a habit.

As a starting point, meditation provides a timeout from activity, allowing you to focus inwardly, rest, and recover. While it may feel like you're doing nothing, you are, in fact, actively training your mind. You can step back from the 24/7 frantic pace of daily life, consciously unwind, and observe what's going on inside. It just takes practise.

Meditation and mindfulness uncover your subconscious biases that lead to poor judgement and bad decisions. They allow you to see the positive lifestyle choices that can drive away negativity in your life. They help you to observe more objectively what you are doing so you can consciously choose healthy habits and let go of unhealthy ones.

Our senses make the world come alive when we're awake in our bodies. It's a truly magnificent experience to discover wisdom, creativity, and love as we relax and awaken through the magnificence of our flesh and being. Even better, it's free! And within our control.

We are all busy being busy, but the best part about meditation and mindfulness is that you can start right now. For only ten minutes a day, you can start developing a healthy habit. Of course, we need skills to know how to do it and a framework to be more mindful.

Meditation helps with that framework, familiarising us with the present. We need to think about our approach to get the most from it. Meditation helps you to step back and see your thoughts and emotions without judgement. It's about focusing your mind on relaxing, allowing you to see things from a different perspective. While we cannot change things that happen to us throughout life, we can change how we perceive our experiences. You don't need to burn a heap of incense, and you don't even have to sit cross-legged on the floor. You genuinely only need to find your ten minutes and step away from everything other than the present moment by surrendering to the now, increasing your focus, and finding clarity.

Don't get me wrong – I use a lot of external tools to help stimulate my senses and relax my mind. My techniques vary and include using essential oils, relaxing music, and a biofeedback headband that reads my breath, posture, and brainwaves, but these were only added to my practice once I mastered the art of switching off. And yes, it is an art form.

Learning to engage with your thoughts, emotions, and external environment is always the most accessible place to start when creating a mindful habit. Like anything new, it just takes time and practise.

MEDITATION STEPS

So, now that you know why, it's time to learn how and get started!

1. Don't overthink it

Many people feel that they can't meditate because it seems so complex and inaccessible. In truth, meditation is precisely the opposite of that! You start with some basic principles you can use anywhere, and, as you practise, you'll improve over time.

There's no need to go in perfectly, so get out of your head and start!

2. Pick your spot

Take a seat somewhere peaceful and quiet. You should feel comfortable enough to sit still for the allotted time but maintain good posture.

3. Decide on your session length

Meditation requires you to sit reasonably still and keep your mind from running away with random thoughts, so it's worth starting with short time segments. Five minutes a day is a good start.

Increase your session length when it feels right.

4. Become conscious of your body

As you start your meditation practice, remember how your body feels. Take the time to assess each body part.

Where are you holding tension? Try to breathe this tension away as you notice it.

Where are you feeling pain? Let your breath deliver healing oxygen to your body, and visualise the pain easing.

Where do you feel good? Savour this feeling as you breathe in and out.

5. Become conscious of your breath

Now that you've checked in with your body, releasing tension and pain where you could, take some time to follow your breath in and out.

Notice how your lungs feel energised with each new breath and how this energy spreads into your body.

6. Deal with your wandering mind

After you've checked in with yourself and focussed on your breathing for some time, it is almost inevitable that your mind will wander. This is the step where many people give up, thinking they can't do it right. The truth is it happens to everyone.

Sometimes we notice our minds wandering at the beginning of a thought, and sometimes we've gone down a five-minute rabbit hole of a fiery, imaginary conversation with the annoying co-worker!

It doesn't matter when you notice, just push pause as soon as you do. Now return to mindfully seeing your breathing.

Over time, your ability to retain focus will improve, benefitting your meditation and your whole life.

7. Finish your session gently

When it's time to finish up, transition back to your day slowly.

Start by becoming more conscious of the things outside your body surrounding you:

* What can you hear?   * What can you smell?

When you're ready, gently open your eyes and notice your surroundings. Ease back into your daily tasks – maybe have a glass of water or a quick walk in the sunshine to make the most of your calmer mindset.

Loz Lesson

To help you create a regular mindfulness practice, download and complete **Take 10** and start working towards building this simple yet effective habit into your morning routine.

TAKE 10
MORNING ROUTINE
MINDFULNESS & MEDITATION

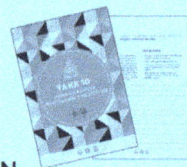

DOWNLOAD YOUR TAKE 10 **lozlife.com/book-take-10**

SLEEP IS WHAT DREAMS ARE MADE OF

Let me be clear – sleep is freaking important. Rest is where we spend about a third of our lives, but most of us don't put enough energy into improving it. Is a lack of sleep limiting your momentum?

Galen, a Greek philosopher and physician from the Roman Empire, suggested that, when awake, the juice from our brains flows out to the rest of our body, making it work. He believed that the brain dries up as the juices flow to the other parts of our bodies, but the fluid then returns while we sleep, thus rehydrating the brain and refreshing the mind.[13] That sounds ridiculous, but was Galen at least correct in his logic?

Based on my experience, resting deeply clears my mind and when I don't sleep, my mind becomes clouded. It's impossible to perpetuate momentum if your sleep is suboptimal.

So many people suffer from sleep deprivation, and our modern lives condition us to have poor sleep habits. Blue light, stimulants, lack of sun exposure throughout the day, and inadequate nutritional intake all contribute to terrible sleep. I don't know about you, but I got sick and tired of being sick and tired!

When was the last time you woke up feeling well-rested? If you're like many people, I bet it was a while ago. Here are my simple tips for sleeping better:

* **You want to aim for seven to nine hours of quality sleep** each night, so reverse engineer the time you need to be in bed by working backwards from when you need to wake up. You will want to use a sleep-tracking device to help you see the quantity and quality of the sleep you are – or aren't – getting.

* **Get some sunshine** during the day or invest in a far infrared light if you live somewhere with frequent overcast weather. This technology has many proven health benefits related to sleep and general wellbeing.[14]

* **Enjoy soothing chamomile tea** after dinner. Apigenin, an antioxidant found in the chamomile flower, is a natural remedy to help with anxiety and can assist with initiating sleep.

* **Avoid television, computers, smartphones,** and other stimulating electronic devices within two hours of bedtime. These devices produce blue light that disrupts your ability to sleep well by turning on the parts of your brain that keep you wired (but tired). Don't fall prey to the late-night scroll hole – read a book instead. If it sounds almost impossible, consider investing in some yellow- or red-tinted blue-blocking glasses that will turn all those blue lights into a less destructive colour so they have a minimal impact on your circadian rhythm.

* **Turn off your wi-fi** before you go to bed. Wireless devices emit constant electromagnetic fields (EMFs), and studies have shown that EMF exposure during sleep can alter brain physiology.[15]

* Once you're in bed, **stop checking your clock.** If you need an alarm to wake up, buy an old-school one so you can keep that phone out of the bedroom.

✳ Use some quality lavender oil on your pillow or **diffuse a relaxing blend of essential oils** in your bedroom. Oils really are such a kick-arse tool.

✳ **Try completing a full-body progressive relaxation** exercise while you're lying in bed. I always do this and end up falling asleep before I'm even finished. You might want to check out my 21-Day Meditation Challenge in the next Loz Lesson.

You'll be surprised by how much creating a consistent, quality sleep ritual with these small but simple activities will change the quality of your rest.

CLIENT STORY – MINDSET IS KEY

When someone has a difficult relationship with sleep, the cause may be physical, mental, or often a combination of the two. Frequently, the solution involves undoing a whole bunch of unhealthy habits and replacing them with some that are more productive. It all comes down to mindset.

Steve's sleep was terrible. Not only did he struggle to fall asleep, but he was waking up at 2 am every day and could not fall back asleep. On average, Steve was only clocking about four hours of shut-eye per night! His brain fog was preventing him from getting any exercise in, and he felt like a hamster on a wheel, burning out every day, unable to recharge. Steve blamed his poor sleep on his age. He had just turned 52.

We met at a business networking event, where he was dosed to the eyeballs with energy drinks and had already smashed three full-strength beers by the time we got chatting. He was in an executive management position at a large engineering company and travelled a lot for work. He was married with no kids and a self-confessed workaholic.

Steve overheard me chatting with someone else at the event about the concept of Handbrake Habits. His ears pricked up when I mentioned how unlocking one habit will incidentally unlock others.

After a brief chat about his crappy sleep and workaholic tendencies, Steve realised that he wasn't actually overly mindful of what he was eating, his posture, his hydration, or his breathing. We arranged a time to catch up again for a discovery chat.

A week later, Steve and I hopped on a Zoom call to help him identify simple yet key areas of his habits that we could easily adjust so he could gain more mental clarity. Using a simple survey, we uncovered that many of his workaholic traits derived from coping strategies he developed during his childhood to earn the love and respect of his father. He learnt that working hard as a hyper achiever gained him love and respect, but this sabotaging coping mechanism was no longer actually serving him. His father had passed away many years ago, yet Steve was still exhibiting traits from decades of trying to earn that same respect. At work, he would always stay back late, often taking his work home, where it would interfere with quality time with his wife. Being on the computer late at night was interfering with his circadian rhythm. He was finding that at around 10 pm, he was hanging for a late-night snack, which usually consisted of half a block of chocolate and ice cream. As you can see, poor sleep was simply a symptom of a longer chain of other detrimental habits that, with some slight tweaking, could be easily adjusted.

With weekly Fab-U Loz coaching, Steve learnt to delegate more work, automate tasks that he was repeating daily, eliminate work that wasn't actually conducive to his success, and engineer more time at the end of the night to be off his screen. On nights where he had deadlines to meet, we implemented some hacks, such as using red-coloured lights and tinted glasses, to mitigate the impact the blue light emitting screens were having on his sleep cycle. Steve started going to bed 15 minutes earlier, which turned into 30 minutes, 45 minutes, an hour, and, finally, two hours earlier. Because he was getting to bed earlier and allowing himself to wind down before bed, he found his sleep was deeper, more restful, and less interrupted. As a result, his morning energy boomed, and he decided to start running around the neighbourhood every day, like he did when he was in his 30s.

Without even really thinking about it, Steve was able to set clear goals for himself, and, as a consequence, his fulfilment at work improved, as did his performance, focus, confidence, and productivity, which rubbed off on his team and his wife. He now spends weekends hiking and bike riding socially.

VOLUNTARY SIMPLICITY

Henry Walden Thoreau popularised the philosophy of voluntary simplicity in the late 1800s. The concept dates back to 300 BC when Epicurus, a Greek philosopher, advocated for moderation in all things. The basis of voluntary simplicity is to practise respect towards others and harness connection with nature around us and our planet. It is about choosing to live life with compassion and thoughtfulness.

As you may realise by now, I enjoy life, but I actually owe a lot of my enjoyment to the fact that I have embraced the concept of voluntary simplicity. I am thankful that everyone's values differ and change, yet they all come from similar principles and emotions of respect, integrity, peace, joy, health, security, and love.

To simplify things in your life and be happier, try these methods!

1. Learn something new

Become inspired by reading a book, listening to a podcast, or watching TV documentaries. Enrich your mind by seeing how other people live, their challenges, and how they survive. See if you can change your life to reflect what you learn.

2. Practise being kind

Kindness is contagious: once you start, others around you will follow. Don't forget to be kind to yourself too. So important – and not always easy.

3. List who is essential to you

Do you find time to spend with important people in your circle of influence? If not, why not? In your process, with whom should you be spending more time? Why not call them now? Life is short! That's a fact.

4. Don't do so much

For many of us, saying "no" can be challenging if we constantly worry about other people's opinions. The trouble is that we become overwhelmed and resentful by saying "yes" out of guilt or perceived expectation from others. Every time we say "yes" to something or someone, we are saying "no" to something or someone else (usually ourselves), and our sanity can sometimes suffer as a consequence.

Perhaps you could say "not yet" and spend that time with someone on your list. Think before you say "yes."

5. Engage with digital media consciously

Be aware of what a time suck TV, social media, and other forms of digital entertainment can be. With regular tech, advertising is aimed to make us feel like we need something more or different and sets unrealistic expectations for us, sometimes without us even realising it. Try to engage with things you can learn from instead – maybe start with books, people, and nature.

6. Know the difference between needs and wants

When buying something, before picking it up, ask yourself, "Do I need this, or do I just want this?" Asking the right questions allows us to be mindful of our purchases. More items do not mean more happiness.

7. Stop multitasking

Do yourself a favour and do one thing at a time. I guarantee your mind will thank you. Regularly, consider one thing you could do now, today, tomorrow, this week, this month, and this year so other items may be deemed easier or even rendered unnecessary. This isn't easy, and we have been taught that multitasking is a skill to master. I happen to think the opposite.

8. Read a book

Read a book that helps you learn. There are many inspirational books to choose from – think about personal development books or memoirs. If you can't sit down to read, consider an audiobook or podcast. I love autobiographical books or texts on self-development. Titles such as *The Subtle Art of Not Giving a F*ck* by Mark Manson, *The ONE Thing* by Gary Keller and Jay Papasan, *The Breakthrough Experience* by Dr John Demartini, or something by Tony Robbins may tickle your fancy.

If books aren't your thing, why not listen to a podcast? There are so many brilliant ones available! Check out the Further Resource Recommendations section at the back of this book for my favourites.

9. Have a tech detox

Remember, in the recent past, we managed to live entirely without our smartphones, tablets, and laptops. A crazy thought. Regular breaks from technology provide us with space to engage in tech-free activities, which are often healthier and more fulfilling.

10. Practise meditation or mindfulness

After reading this chapter, you may want to practise mindfulness, not being swept up by your feelings or thoughts. You'll learn how to acknowledge them and not react, stay present in the moment, and change how you experience your life. Walking can assist with this process, or perhaps you can sit quietly for a moment and use a guided meditation app to help you find inner calm. My favourite app is Muse, and I use it with a high-tech, real-time, biofeedback headband that reads my brainwaves. Sounds cool, and it is. Alternatively, Headspace and The Breathing App are easy meditation tools that can assist you in quieting your mind.

Loz Lesson

To help you learn how to switch off your brain,
try my **21-Day Meditation Challenge**.

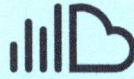

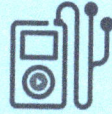

**21 DAY
MEDITATION CHALLENGE**

DOWNLOAD YOUR MEDITATION CHALLENGE **lozlife.com/book-meditation**

11. Channel your green thumb

Do you have somewhere you can grow or keep plants? If you have space for a garden, you may learn to develop the foods you love. If space is limited, use your balcony, patio, or windowsill to grow herbs as a simple start. Nothing is more satisfying than watching a little dried-up, hard lump – the seed – turn into a plant, providing food. It's pretty freaking magical!

12. Become a conscious shopper

Buying a product that is kinder to our environment can make you feel good, whether it be recycled packaging, biodegradable, or organic. Next time you shop, why not purchase a brand that you know is environmentally conscious, say, from a company that plants trees or uses renewable energy? Supporting small businesses by choosing a local supplier is also a great way to impact your community by consciously shopping. Shop local, people!

SELF-CARE VS. SELF-SOOTHING

We talk a lot about 'self-care', about the importance of taking time out just for you. Time to relax, recharge, and refocus. As we all know, sometimes it's easier said than done. Life gets in the way; kids get in the way, and work gets in the way. Days, weeks, and months – even years – roll by, and suddenly you realise you can't recall the last time you had time just for you.

At the other end of the self-care spectrum, you often make time for self-care. But is it self-care or self-soothing you're committed to? As I found out recently, there's a difference, and that difference may come down to treating yourself versus healing yourself.

I had the pleasure of attending an International Women's Day event in 2022, where a friend spoke about the definition of self-care and alerted us all to the fact that, while we think we're taking good care of ourselves, often we are actually self-soothing. What's the difference? Well, it comes down to being proactive versus reactive.

Self-soothing is reactive. It's retreating from the world when the going gets tough and taking time to hide away and heal. Sometimes it's absolutely needed, but it's not self-care. Self-care is proactive. It prioritises your mental health and deliberately schedules positive activities just for you, no matter how you feel. Self-care is a preventative approach.

So, you've had a bad week, and you need a little 'me time' away from the world. You grab a bottle of ice-cold sav blanc and a block of chocolate and snuggle up on the couch under the doona to binge-watch Netflix. No judgement here. I get it! The trouble is, this is not self-care. This is self-soothing. It's a momentary, transient fix that, in the long term, can be detrimental to your health (physical, emotional, and mental).

Committing to self-care is about showing up for yourself. It's about creating a proactive, preventative plan.

Maybe it's taking a long, hot bath with a good book. Perhaps it's taking a walk while listening to an audiobook or podcast. Possibly it's booking a float or a massage. Maybe it's doing a gym class or learning to paint. Only you can decide what self-care activities are best for you.

I understand that Netflix, a bottle of wine, and a block of choc can be a great solution. And it might be, at that moment, as it can distract you from your problems… momentarily. But it's not a good choice for your body in the long run. You are sugar-coating your problems with chocolate, then washing them down with wine. We've literally all done it!

However, genuine, positive self-care is about doing something that feels good and good for you. See the difference? Let's look at it another way. When craving self-care, is it because you are running away from something terrible or towards something good? It's an interesting question, isn't it? I challenge you to ask yourself this question next time you're about to veg out on the couch with the doona, wine, chocolate, and the 'flix after a bad day.

Self-soothing tends to be related to running away, whereas self-care is generally a more positive approach towards living a better life so you don't need to self-soothe so often. So many of my clients have spent far too long running away from the bad rather than focussing on running towards the good, especially when it comes to their diet, weight, and fitness. But, together, we create a proactive, preventative plan to help them achieve their weight loss goals. A plan that includes genuine self-care. Because, like the ad says, you're worth it.

You're freaking awesome!

DEALING WITH GRIEF

I want to talk about grief for a minute. Because, let's face it, it can be pretty bloody overwhelming. Grief is a natural response to loss. It's the emotional suffering you feel when something or someone you love is taken away.

The pain of loss can often feel devastating, heartbreaking, overwhelming, and terrifying. You may experience difficult and unexpected emotions, from shock or anger to disbelief, guilt, and profound sadness. The pain of grief can also disrupt your physical health, making it difficult to sleep, eat, or even think straight. These are normal reactions to loss – the more significant the loss, the more intense your grief will be.

When you lose someone or something you love, it's hard to imagine life without them. Every loss comes with pain and adjustments we need to make.

It's important to note that while we usually associate grief with death, it can hit hard for various reasons: from divorce or a relationship breakdown, health issues, losing a job, losing money, a miscarriage, death of a pet, a loved one's serious illness, loss of a friendship, loss of safety after trauma… the list goes on.

I don't believe you get over the loss; instead, you must work out how to accept it. I have faced a lot of grief in my time, from Brian's suicide to dealing with the loss of my relationship with my father. It doesn't get easier, but I have gotten better at identifying the stages and knowing how to best move through them.

I have responded to grief in all kinds of ways, and not all of them positively. I've struggled with depression and eating disorders. I've shut people I love out.

I have learnt that you naturally learn how to grieve by grieving. Creating positive habits around how you deal with grief helps with the process. Positive habits, like exercise and seeking regular help from a qualified professional, can help break the cycle of suffering.

Grief hits hard in unexpected ways. It's an organic process unique to you and to each situation. The key is to be conscious and aware so you're always learning and moving forward to embrace it and to push through it. Momentum is key.

Before we talk about the seven steps of grief, it's important to note that this isn't a neat, step-by-step process. Nope. Best to interpret the stages loosely and expect a lot of variation. Sometimes it's a case of three steps forward and four back. The steps can occur out of order. However, this is an excellent guide to knowing what to expect. There is no 'normal' when it comes to grief.

For some, there is quite an extensive mourning process that comes with the various stages of grief. This is why grief symptoms can be a significant indicator to someone about what stage of grief and loss they are currently going through. So, what are the seven stages of grief?

1. Shock and denial

You will probably react to learning of the loss with numbed disbelief. You may deny the reality of the loss at some level to avoid the pain. The shock provides emotional protection from being overwhelmed all at once. This may last for weeks.

This type of grief is probably one of the biggest and most important stages that people go through once they start processing the grief after suicide – a stage I can attest to.

Emotions during this time could include mourning, sadness, confusion, and discomfort.

2. Pain and guilt

As the shock wears off, it is replaced with the suffering of unbeliev-able pain. Although excruciating and almost unbearable, you must experience the pain fully and not hide it, avoid it, or escape it with alcohol or drugs.

You may feel guilty or remorseful over things you did or didn't do with your loved one. Life feels chaotic and scary during this phase.

Emotions during this time could include sadness, guilt, despera-tion, and betrayal.

3. Anger and bargaining

Frustration gives way to anger, and you may lash out and lay unwar-ranted blame for the death on someone else. Please try to control this, as permanent damage to your relationships may result. This is not a time for the release of bottled-up emotion. You may rail against fate, asking, "Why me?" You may also try to bargain in vain with the powers that be for a way out of your despair: "I will never drink again if you just bring him back!"

If you haven't already, considering grief counselling is a good idea at this stage.

Emotions felt during this time could include anger, resentment, bargaining, and stubbornness.

4. 'Depression', reflection, and loneliness

Just when your friends may think you should be getting on with your life, a long period of sad reflection will likely overtake you. This is a normal stage of grief, so do not be 'talked out of it' by well-meaning outsiders. Encouragement from others is not helpful to you during this stage of grieving.

During this time, you finally realise the true magnitude of your loss, and it depresses you. You may isolate yourself on purpose, reflect on things you did with your lost one, and focus on memories of the past. You may sense feelings of emptiness or despair.

Emotions felt during this time could include heaviness, despair, and frustration.

5. The upward turn

As you adjust to life without your loved one, your life becomes calmer and more organised. Your physical symptoms lessen, and your 'depression' begins to lift slightly.

This is the part of the grieving process where you'll start to see the light at the end of the tunnel. It's a middle ground of all the grief symptoms that you'll go through, but it's one you can build upon.

Emotions felt during this time could include strength, motivation, and awakening.

6. Reconstruction and working through

As you become more functional, your mind starts working again, and you will find yourself seeking realistic solutions to problems posed by life without your loved one. You will begin to work on practical and financial issues and reconstruct yourself and your life without him or her.

Emotions felt during this time could include inspiration, determination, and refreshment.

7. Acceptance and hope

During this, the last of the seven stages in this grief model, you learn to accept and deal with the reality of your situation. Acceptance does not necessarily mean instant happiness.

Given the pain and turmoil you have experienced, you can never return to the carefree, untroubled you that existed before this tragedy – but you will find a way forward. You will start to look ahead and plan things for the future.

Eventually, you can think about your lost loved one without pain. Sadness, yes! But the wrenching pain will be gone. You will again anticipate some good times to come and even find joy again in the experience of living. You have made it through the seven stages of grief.

Emotions felt during this time could include hope, comfort, relaxation, security.

For me, grief is still a part of my every day. I will always miss Brian immensely. It's an ongoing journey and one that I embrace.

By learning how you best deal with grief, and the seven stages, you can better mitigate the negative impacts next time. Because sorry, friends, there will always be a next time.

REFINING NOT DEFINING

I am always learning. I love it because it helps me grow and become a better human, and I am open to all kinds of perspectives and theories, no matter their origin.

Recently, I came across an Eastern perspective on identity that I want to share.

Firstly, let's talk about how the Western world understands identity and personality formation. Long story short, we believe we are born a blank canvas and our personalities and identities are formed through our experiences and learnings. Layer upon layer. Makes sense.

However, the Eastern world takes a different approach. This culture believes that we are born like a rough block of jade. Every challenge we face – grief, trauma, love, loss – chips away at that jade, inch by inch.

Eventually, the authentic you will be revealed. It was there all along, your essence, hidden away in the core of that rough block of jade. Waiting to be discovered. Waiting to be refined, as opposed to defined.

That's the difference between the two philosophies. The East believes we begin our lives with an identity refined as we live. The West believes we start our lives with nothing and it's defined as we live life.

Refined vs. defined. I like Eastern philosophy, as it reflects my 'me-search' quest to refine myself, learn more, and mould and shape myself daily.

MOVING TOWARDS A MORE SIMPLIFIED LIFE

Hands up, who feels like their life is super complicated? Yep, I hear ya! It might be time to dial it back a bit and simplify things.

I am not saying that simplifying your life will be easy, but it will make you mindful of what you say and do. Living a simpler life makes you feel good and helps make for a better world. Pretty cool, huh?

Despite the many daily challenges, it feels incredibly satisfying to live my values more broadly by tapping into simplicity.

Leonardo da Vinci once said, "Simplicity is the ultimate sophistication."

I always strive to do more and give more, and I love inspiring others to do the same, but I regularly ask myself questions about whether my actions or thoughts serve me at this moment. Am I considerate to the planet? And, equally as important, am I kind to myself? If I do just one thing today, will this task make other tasks easier or unnecessary? Just by asking these simple questions, I not only choose to do something to make my life simpler and more productive, but I also consider each action with deep gratitude.

Let's talk about gratitude. Such a powerful practice.

Gratitude is by far the healthiest of all human emotions. No matter how good or bad you feel, you must wake up each day thankful for your life because happiness is a choice. I have learnt that life is a series of thousands of tiny miracles, and I am starting to notice them daily – because I look for them. Although I never wanted kids of my own, now that I'm a stepmum and stepgrandparent, I'm thankful for my struggle up to this point in my life because, without it, I wouldn't have stumbled across the opportunities to embrace my inherent maternal instinct. To see a child experience the sensations of something as simple as the beach for the first time is breathtaking. God, I adore the little people in my life! Yes, I am grateful for them.

So, start each day with a grateful heart because the real secret to having it all is knowing that you already do. Read that line twice!

THE POWER OF VISUALISATION

Ever wished you could meditate but use the excuse that it's "too hard" because you can't shut off your mind? Mindfulness and meditation can help you tap into your deepest desires by living in the moment. You can do it!

When you take the time to be silent and slow down, you can more clearly visualise what you want to create. Personally, my most brilliant and vivid ideas come to me when I'm in a deep meditative state (or even when I'm facedown on a massage table getting acupuncture… *boom*… instant ideas).

If you're like most people, when your mind is full and busy, it is like a stormy sea, with frothing waves thrashing onto the shore. If we take time out to live in the now and make the time to meditate, the storm disappears; the tide calmly washes over the beach, and the water is more transparent. In short, our mind becomes focused, calm, and present. Who doesn't want that?

Mindfulness practice can help you visualise what you most want to manifest by providing a brain space for creation. It's incredibly cool.

HOW CAN I START PRACTISING MINDFULNESS?

Your body and brain are not built to run in the constant overdrive of modern living and multitasking. Yet, we do it. Well, we try. You were designed to engage in a specific activity, then to rest and recover from what you've achieved. During that downtime, your body integrates all you have experienced and heals any cellular damage sustained.

Biohacks, like sleep and exercise trackers, sequential compression devices, infrared light therapy, or massage can help with physical recovery. These are very useful, but your systems will eventually go haywire if you don't honour the synergistic balance between activity and recovery.

Mindfulness can help us feel better and calmer and increase our self-awareness. Ultimately, that awareness helps us care for ourselves and shapes us to be the best versions of ourselves. If you can practise mindfulness regularly, it can become a tool to discover if your work is actually supporting you.

Mindfulness can be your guide and can help you choose your work direction. Think about what you do in a single day – how often do you feel balanced or stressed?

Balance is excellent so if you feel it when you undertake daily tasks, you should acknowledge it. What about right now, as you're reading this? Do you feel in balance? If you do, stop and feel it for a moment. Honour this feeling and enjoy it. Yay, you!

We tend to be conditioned to think stress is wrong. Still, there are two distinct variations of stress, as differentiated by endocrinologist Hans Selye in 1975. The first type, *eustress*, is conducive to balance and usually enhances our function by giving us a feeling of fulfilment. An example of eustress would be participating in competitive sport, where it's simultaneously challenging and rewarding. The second type is *distress*.[16] Well, it's the kind that causes people to end up having mental breakdowns and can lead to illness. Are you feeling uneasy or feeling tense right at this moment? It's good to acknowledge your state. Don't judge yourself. It's not helpful. Instead, be mindful of what your body is doing and how it warns you that it's starting to feel stressed.

With either type of stress – eustress or distress – stop and think about what these feelings make you mindful of. Obviously, be aware of your reactions.

Mindfulness at Work

If work seems to cause you regular distress – as it once did for me – you can ask yourself a few questions to help you become more aware of being mindful during specific tasks:

* Do I feel **more stressed** when I am working on writing assignments?

* When I speak about particular topics, **does my voice change**?

* What tasks **increase my tension**?

Sometimes, the prospect of specific tasks can instigate a deep, emotional response. Be mindful of when you feel certain emotions and take note of what you are doing at the time by asking:

* What am I doing when I **feel joyful**?

* What is it that **stops my flow** of enjoyment?

* When do I **feel small** or **limited**?

When you start to grow your awareness around your mindfulness and are cognisant of your feelings and what tasks you are undertaking at the time, it can be helpful to ask yourself:

* Do I **want more** of these things?

* Do I **want to rid** myself of these things?

* Now that I am mindful of these things, how do I **make the change**?

* If I do make the change in both my work and my lifestyle, **what will occur**?

While making these changes, be mindful of how you feel. It's pretty incredible what you will start to notice.

SETTING GOALS

Are you a goal setter and achiever? How many goals have you set throughout your life? How many have you followed through on? Goals, such as writing a book, going on a magical holiday, saving money, making money, decluttering our life, and cool ones like losing weight and getting fit, are achievable dreams. Still, they tend to stay as dreams unless we can create strategic plans to make them a reality. Because a goal without a plan is just a wish!

Now, as a business owner, organising is my thing. I am always goal setting, thinking big, planning, strategising, and mapping out my dreams to make them *goals*, but I don't believe I was always like this. I used to be a serial dream setter, but now I'm a goal-setting legend if I do say so myself. I make lists, use Post-it notes and project management apps (such as Trello and Asana), strategically colour-code my calendar with highlighters, and fill my walls with printed plans and hand-scrawled mind maps. Seriously, I have more stationery than Officeworks. I also have a stack of affirmation decks and quotation cards, and I pull out random ones daily to help me stay focused. Honestly, I'm an inspiration addict!

Now that I've created a lifestyle that most people dream of, I immerse myself in learning by attending workshops to thrive and grow. I love attending seminars, listening to podcasts, reading books, and undertaking online courses. Many of my goals come to fruition when I learn new information. Remember, goals can sometimes be simplified and achieved by learning something fresh daily.

Oh, and I also surround myself with kick-arse, inspiring people.

BUILDING A 'LEARNING-INSPIRATION ENGINE'

Sometimes, I cannot believe how much I fit into one day. I know I'm a bit of an energetic freak. I help my clients, create new content, write, think, run my business, attend meetings and events, care for my dog, love my husband, talk to my mum every second day, try to keep up with friends, exercise regularly, eat healthily – the list goes on. All good, right?

Well, in the beginning, after a lot of soul-searching and journalling, I realised I wasn't getting the results I wanted. I wasn't achieving my most important goals. I was always 'busy being busy', but I continuously found that I was not focusing on the actions that would help me achieve my big, delicious goals because I was constantly distracted by other tasks. I had too many things on my to-do list. Oh, look… another shiny object!

Eventually, it became overwhelming, and I was so focused on maintaining a state of 'busyness' that I had no time to stop and think. I was spread way too thin and gave no regard to how I felt while doing all this stuff. Half the time, I was doing things for the sake of doing stuff. With so many unrelated goals, I became overloaded. Sound familiar?

So, how do we align our actions with our goals and achieve the results we seek?

Firstly, fewer is always better. Three words to remember – fewer, bigger, better. That's how I try to live my life now. Because it's a mathematical equation: you still have only 100 percent of yourself to give… if you spread yourself too thin, lots of things will get a small amount of attention. Focus breeds success.

To succeed and grow, it's essential to realise that you cannot do everything alone. The most successful people surround themselves with a team to help them.

We must sort out the obsolete obstacles if we want to play to our strengths and achieve goals aligned with our highest priorities and values. The five ways to do this are through:

1. **Delegating** tasks to others if the job does not align with your highest values. For example, I use a bookkeeper, graphic designer, and virtual assistant to help me complete tasks that may take me a long time if I do them on my own. I can't do it all!

2. **Automating** processes using technology and computer applications. For example, when I buy things for my business, I use an app on my phone to take a photo of the receipt at the time of purchase, and the app stores this receipt digitally. This saves me from manually entering receipts into my accounting software at tax time. I'm really not superb at that stuff…

3. **Collaborating** with others who can help you brainstorm ideas or provide another opinion. For example, I have built a network of like-minded people to call upon when I need help critiquing a goal, plan, or idea. I love catching up with them!

4. **Innovating** or improving processes you have undertaken in the past or even creating brand-new ideas. After every project or task, review and readjust. For example, I realised that many of my clients were struggling to find a meditation program that was easy to follow. I helped them build their confidence by slowly introducing them to mindfulness. As a result, I identified a gap in the market, which led to innovation. I created my 21-Day Meditation Challenge. *ICYMI: Go back to the last Loz Lesson to access this for yourself!*

5. **Eliminating** tasks that rob you of time or may be unnecessary because they won't really add any value to your overall goal. For example, I used to always have my nails done during bodybuilding – it just seemed like the thing to do. This seemingly small activity actually took several hours out of every fortnight. When I eliminated this task from my schedule, I freed up the time to play with my dog and spend more time with my husband. I now get my nails done for special occasions, and I appreciate it a lot more (and save money – bonus!).

When I started to experience burnout, I realised all I had to do was work out which things in my life meant the most – my priorities. I asked myself, "What activities are conducive to achieving my goals because they align with my highest values?" I also asked, "What's the one thing I could do today that would make other things easier or unnecessary?" The answer to these questions will uncover your priorities.

By simply scaling back on a heap of misaligned goals, I could achieve a hell of a lot more and focus on activities that added value to my life. What did that help me to do? Yep. You guessed it. Get the f*ck unstuck!

Only by being far more consistent with daily tasks and commitments could I take a distinct path towards achieving meaningful goals with purposeful intent.

One day, not too long ago, I made it my purpose to spend the rest of my life laughing, celebrating, teaching, connecting, and surrounding myself with incredible, positive people. I aligned how I wanted to feel in my personal life with the goals I wanted to achieve in my business life. This shift from 'busy' to 'fulfilled' allowed me to set myself free of piles of self-imposed egocentric bullshit. And guess what? I am no longer busy being busy.

In a nutshell, success is just a series of small wins and a state of mind. With consistency, moving towards your goal brings about balance and purposeful productivity.

My Advice...

If you haven't found success yet (whatever you define that to be), keep looking. Don't give up. It's 100 percent up to you to design a life you love. Seriously, you will only fail if you give up on yourself. That is an absolute fact. And if you can't support your dreams, how can you expect anyone else to?

If what you're doing, thinking, and feeling doesn't add value and happiness to your life, it doesn't belong there. Chuck it out with the junk mail. Make your dreams happen. Go where you feel vividly alive. Stop holding yourself back because if you aren't happy, know that you are in absolute control and can make a change.

Want to know what's powerful? The fact that wherever you are in your life, that's on you. Okay, depending on how you feel about your life, that might be a bit of a terrifying realisation… that you only have yourself to blame. Yes, that means owning some serious shit.

But, in fantastic news, it also means that you have the power to make any change you want. Today. Right now. To alter the course of your life.

IS YOUR MINDSET HOLDING YOU BACK?

Back in the chapter on momentum, you were prompted to think about what actions you will take right now, tomorrow, next week, next month, next year, and every day for the rest of your life to achieve your ideal lifestyle. Do you have a clear end goal? What does it feel, smell, taste, and look like to accomplish this goal? Can you visualise it as if you've already smashed it? Please write it down, say it aloud, and tell a friend. Make it real!

To succeed, you need to set defined goals (or intentions) to enable you to focus and direct your life. To take control of your direction in life, setting intentions gives you benchmarks to ensure you succeed.

You need to know how to set a goal and not just hold onto ideas as 'dreams' because, unfortunately, things don't just happen. Dreams only work if you do.

Goal setting is a process that starts with defining where you are and where you want to be and strategising, with clear, purposeful steps… and a lot of hard work in between. Yep. Hard work is compulsory, I'm afraid.

Sometimes our mindset is holding us back from setting, and achieving, goals for ourselves. The series of self-perceptions or beliefs about ourselves can influence our behaviour, outlook, and mental attitude. For a lot of people, this can be as simple as the belief that they are either intelligent or unintelligent, lucky or unlucky, or even sick or healthy.

People can generally have a 'fixed mindset' or a 'growth mindset'. Most of us have both but use them differently, depending on the circumstance. For example, a growth mindset might be applied to our job, and a fixed mindset might apply to our general self-esteem.

A growth mindset is characterised by a person believing that their necessary abilities can be developed through hard work and dedication. Talent and brains are only the beginning.

In contrast, a fixed mindset is characterised by those who believe that talent and intelligence are things people are born with and cannot be acquired. These people waste time thinking they are unable to develop these traits. It's a negative way to live. They allow success or failure to define them. Someone with a fixed mindset will consider themselves either intelligent or dumb and will negatively convince themselves there is no way of changing. They will think that they "can't do that" or will make excuses to rationalise failure. Damn you, shitty self-talk!

The key to setting realistic goals is to unlock our mindset patterns and recognise and call ourselves out on our self-sabotaging ways and limiting beliefs. That way, through self-limitation, we can be free of the burdens we place on our own lives.

Remember to be kind to yourself. Always. If you didn't take action on something, go back to your goals and work out why. Perhaps brainstorm an alternative activity that may align with your values but achieve the same outcome.

To summarise this chapter, meditation is an attention-training technique, and mindfulness is a productive attitude for practising this technique. Meditation allows you to practise mindfulness. Meditation and mindfulness give you a deeper understanding of how your mind works and opens your life to your potential for happiness and wellness. They really do help. I promise! When mindful, we can define clear goals and action plans to succeed, as they will come from a place of purpose and intention.

Ultimately, tapping into mindfulness connects you to your health and wellbeing. Mindfulness allows you to focus on your work and identify thoughts and activities that support your efforts to improve the quality of your life. Mindfulness helps you pay attention to your reactions to stressors in your life, work, and among those around you. Yes, people too.

No matter what happens in your life, positivity, patience, and persistence will evoke more energy, initiative, and happiness. A great mindset is about seeing the invisible and feeling the intangible. Deep, I know.

Be strong, be fearless, be beautiful, be you. With the right people to support you, you will believe that anything is possible – and it is.

You know what? I'm grateful that I know who I am. I am certainly not perfect. I am not the most beautiful woman in the world, but I am one of them. My journey continues because I've conquered a lot in my unique Loz way, and I now know how to overcome the rest. Yep, I'm f*cking resilient, but I also work hard to use the right strategies to help me through challenges and adversity.

Ultimately, you, too, are powerful and can achieve anything you put your mind to!

Take the time to be mindful, and create the space to set goals and focus. The more you practise, the more quickly it becomes a routine, and the sooner it transforms into a healthy habit.

Because that's the most powerful thing we can do – create healthy habits.

We are all capable of perfection. We must accept that each moment is already perfect and just waiting for us to seize it. It's all a matter of perspective and mindset. The mind really is a bloody powerful tool.

Using all the strategies outlined in this chapter, you should now better understand how to set that goal you have always wanted to achieve. Feeling how we wish to be can be as simple as taking action to design a path to our success.

Loz Lesson

To help you map your goals, download and complete **SMART Goals**. You might discover that creating a single target makes you feel compelled to make more!

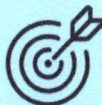

SMART GOALS
THE BUILDING BLOCKS
TO YOUR SUCCESS

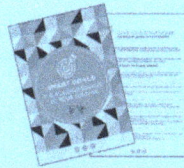

DOWNLOAD YOUR SMART GOALS **lozlife.com/book-smart-goals**

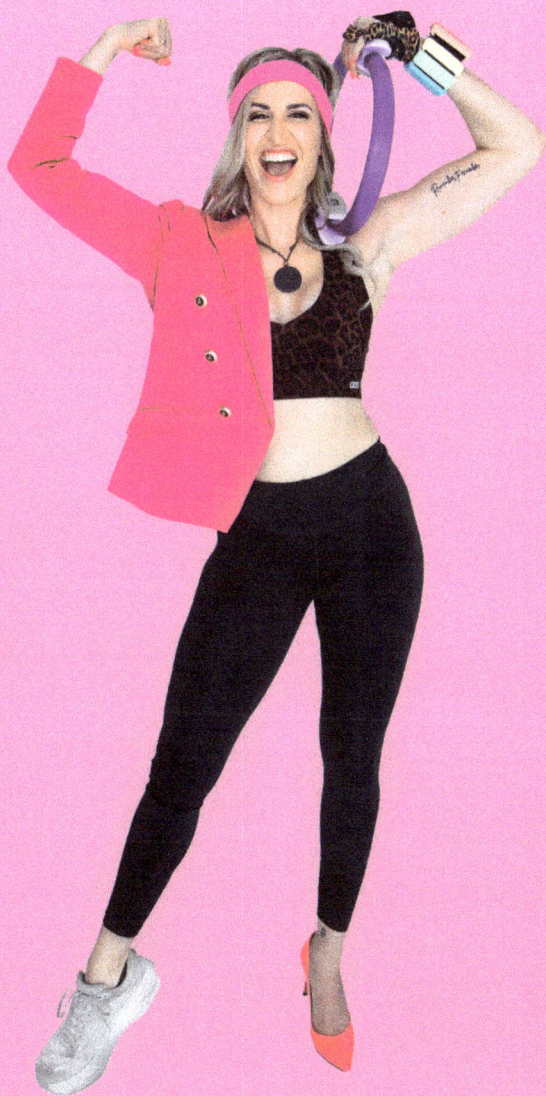

MOVEMENT

Now that you've worked on unlocking your fears, fuelling your body, and creating structured goals, it's time to focus on movement improvement. This is totally non-negotiable. You need to move that body!

I'm often asked, "Do I really need to exercise?"

The short answer is YES! Exercise prevents disease. As an active person, you're statistically less likely to develop osteoporosis, type 2 diabetes, or cardiovascular disease. You're also less likely to suffer from a stroke or develop certain cancers, such as colon and breast cancer. It's scary to consider, but a lack of physical activity is ranked just behind cigarette smoking as a cause of ill health. Shocking, right?!

Mindful improvement of daily movement plays an integral role in helping us regulate our moods and maintain optimal physical health. In essence, regular activity improves the quality of life. Lead yourself to mastery with your body, and your mind will follow. It's that simple yet super powerful.

How many people have endured gruelling 12-week challenges and lost a stack of weight, only to put it all back on in due course and then a bit extra? Yep, I've done it too.

Only some people want to be so fit that they can run a marathon every week. Sure, you may want to avoid scaling Mount Everest. I get that. Optimum movement and mobility mean different things to different people. For someone who's 90 years old, maybe all they want to do is feel 'capable' so they can walk unassisted, wipe their bum, and tie their shoes (because bottom wipers are an actual product, and I have sold many of them in my time!). Essentially, being able to choose the most suitable and effective way to keep your body active as you evolve and mature is critical to maintaining vitality for life – and it is your choice.

Mastering movement and becoming biomechanically efficient will positively affect everything you do in your life. Whether for sports and athletics, overall fitness, or everyday life, action is vital for sustaining a sound body and avoiding injury.

Many people need their movement corrected. Movement improvement habits can only be achieved sustainably once momentum, menu, and mindset outcomes have been reached. Imagine your body as a race car and your mindset as the driver. If you fill the vehicle with suboptimal fuel and aren't thinking straight, chances are you'll drive pretty poorly and probably have a few crashes on the racetrack. Eeek! This is why movement sits so high in my Healthy Habit Hierarchy.

We know from scientific research that oxidative stress and inflammation are at the root of most chronic illnesses. It is not sufficient for your health for me to advise you to "go and eat healthily and exercise." It's neither specific nor meaningful enough for most people to implement. It is crucial to educate the public about their redox status – that is, the ratio between free radicals causing oxidative stress and antioxidants to counteract the pro-oxidants.

Our ability to fight oxidative stress is the most significant determinant of our cellular health. And yes, I'm getting technical, but bear with me. We can have the very best intentions for our health, but the truth is, without understanding how our bodies respond to a specific stimulus, we could be increasing the levels of oxidative stress on our cells.

In its simplest terms, to maintain optimal vitality – aka kick-arse energy – it's essential to integrate consistent movement into our daily routine. If we don't, we suffer from motion starvation, and our bodies will begin to reflect the dysfunctions we create inside, manifested as pain, illness, and structural deficits. Movement is a renewable resource that must be replenished responsibly and continuously.

MOVEMENT FOR OPTIMUM MOBILITY

As a personal trainer, group fitness instructor, and Pilates specialist, I want this chapter to inspire you to move your body in a way that resonates with your soul. That's how I view it. Imagine being able to move freely, with no pain, well into your senior years. How good would that feel?

Humans are the best movers on the planet, and movement patterns are directly correlated to connections between mind, muscle, fascia, and nerves. Functional movement is the ability to move your body using your muscles and joints effortlessly and without pain. Optimal movement requirements differ from one person to the next. As I mentioned earlier in this chapter, for an elderly person, optimal movement may be as simple as the ability to do everyday things. For you and me, optimal movement may be as bold as being physically capable of scaling the world's highest mountains!

You would think your body would just naturally work well, but unfortunately this is often not the case. From birth, you start to build up dominant and weaker muscles. You experience inadequate muscle utilisation, and injury or mishap can further limit your body's capacity to develop reliably. The result – you cannot fully use the ideal form or support to train functional movement systems for whole-body health and fitness. In lay terms, your body doesn't work the way it should.

The human body is designed for movement, but many of us live sedentary lives and often spend long hours in the same position, such as sitting in front of a computer. This lack of movement results in aches and pains, a lack of energy, and, often, obesity. A sedentary lifestyle also prematurely decreases the functional capability of your body. You are probably familiar with the adage 'use it or lose it', which is undoubtedly true for movement and a healthy body. So, what's your excuse for not moving it?

Worldwide, people struggle to manage their weight, and we have developed many strategies that keep it that way. For example, the famous New Year's Eve resolution, which we set with the best intentions, to exercise after the holidays… you know how it goes. By Valentine's Day, those good intentions are long forgotten, and your gym membership is gathering dust.

Understanding how to choose the right type of movement and the most effective way to keep your body functionally active is critical to maintaining vitality for life. As we age, it's essential to recognise that we must evolve our choices of physical activity to match our lifestyle and natural abilities. Many people use the excuse, "Oh, I'm too old for that" when it comes to exercise. Newsflash – you're never too old. Never!

An exercise regimen should take into account your age and health. Even if your body doesn't move as well as it used to, we can certainly exercise our minds. The reality is our bodies don't always cooperate.

Now, you're probably thinking, just how much exercise do you need to do to see the benefits? Simply put, you certainly don't have to train for a marathon. Something as simple as regular stair climbing or walking can be healthy and effective.

All experts agree that exercise needs to be regular and moderately intense, and the guidelines recommend a minimum of 30 minutes of moderate exercise on most days of the week. But how do you know if your exercise is moderate? The best test is to see if you can easily talk while doing the exercise. If you can, you are exercising in the light to moderate range. If your breathing gets in the way of speaking, you know you have increased the intensity. Yay, you!

Using tools, such as electronic activity monitors (Fitbits, smart watches, and so on) and heart rate monitors (for example, Polar) is another simple way to objectively measure the intensity of physical activity and to benchmark yourself for future improvement. Research suggests a positive correlation between the intensity and length of exercise and reduction in risk of coronary conditions.[17] If you don't have access to activity monitors, remember that the more intense and the longer you exercise, the more significant the benefit becomes. Simple really.

Don't worry too much if you are just starting to exercise. Luckily for you, daily light activity is beneficial in preventing obesity and diabetes. New research shows that sitting for long periods can increase blood glucose levels, even if you exercise.[18] For this reason, just staying active and complementing your 30 minutes of exercise with regular light activity is a sure path to greater vitality. Exercise is always a good thing.

My advice

Always check with a health professional before ramping up any movement beyond 'moderate', particularly if you're new to exercise. They can design an exercise plan for you, which will help avoid injuries usually caused by exercising too quickly or too much.

CHOOSING THE BEST EXERCISE FOR YOU

Why is it that some people see exercise as extremely difficult, but it's almost second nature for others? In fact, they love it.

Deciding what sort of physical activity suits your lifestyle isn't as challenging as you think. To help you choose, it's vital to understand the different categories of movement we can use to keep us active and healthy.

CLIENT STORY – A TAILORED APPROACH TO MOVEMENT

When it comes to movement, I have coached clients of all types and abilities, and working around physical limitations and other constraints is a big part of that.

Bridget was seven months postpartum and was struggling to find a consistent workout schedule now that she had a baby. Before becoming a mum, Bridget was training five days a week at a local CrossFit gym and, since having her child, really missed working out. She dabbled in Pilates but found it gave her back pain. After giving birth, she tried to go back to CrossFit but didn't have the consistency in her schedule to train like she used to. She also hurt her shoulder doing some lifts and was scared to go back to high-intensity training. Plus, when she did any high-impact jumping activities, she would pee her pants. She now had constant headaches from tight shoulders, and breastfeeding a hungry bub was even more challenging because of her posture.

Bridget and I met at a team building day her workplace hosted, where I ran a hybrid group exercise and relaxation session that included elements of Pilates, flow work, breathing, and mindful meditation. During the session, I taught the group how to self-palpate to ensure they activated their pelvic floor and deep core muscles to stabilise their spine and actually use the right muscles when they exercised.

At the end of the session, Bridget approached me and told me that no one had ever explained how to self-palpate, or even how to breathe properly (which, as a Pilates instructor, I'm always surprised to hear). She said that for the very first time, she experienced zero back pain with the Pilates exercises and actually felt her core working. Bridget decided to hire me as a one-on-one coach for a few sessions to help her create a more structured exercise program that would fit her new life as a mum.

During our first session, I undertook a movement screening with Bridget, and it was clear that she had poor pelvic strength and rounded shoulders due to overuse of her upper trap muscles from many years of CrossFit. She was very quadricep dominant in her physical build (that is, the fronts of her thighs were very muscular compared to the backs of her thighs), and she hated her flat butt. Although looking good was important to her, Bridget's main fitness goal was to be able to be an active mum as her child grew. She planned to have more kids in a few years, and her primary focus was to feel better and create a new active lifestyle that could include her partner and her child, without her feeling like she was holding them back.

I commenced Bridget on a Pilates-based posture program to help open her chest, turn off her overused trap muscles (by balancing out her upper back), and strengthen her pelvic floor – we worked specifically on developing her gluteal muscles. Using the principles of Pilates (posture, breathing, and core control), she was able to relieve her headaches and improve her continence challenges. Bridget also discovered a love for triathlons and competed in her first competition when her daughter turned 18 months.

THE SEVEN DIMENSIONS OF FITNESS

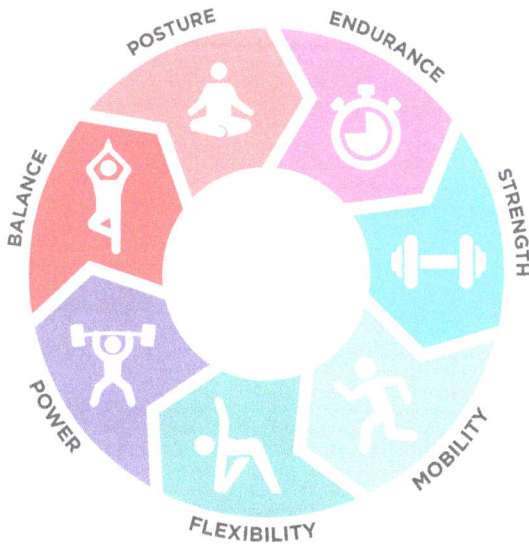

There are several types of movement to consider when planning your fitness journey. These include:

1. Balance
2. Posture
3. Endurance
4. Strength
5. Power
6. Flexibility
7. Mobility

Working on all seven types across the three fundamental categories of cardiovascular exercise, resistance training, and flexibility is recommended for long-term physical advantage, emphasising cardiovascular activity.

Cardiovascular Exercise

This type of exercise is anything that raises your heart rate. Primarily, your level of cardiovascular movement is considered the most significant predictor of mortality, and this type of exercise has the highest impact on your ability to undertake everyday activities.

The recommendation is to engage in cardiovascular exercise between three to five times a week, either 20 minutes at high intensity or 45 minutes at a lower intensity. Practise this type of exercise by including nose breathing where possible, as this will increase oxygen uptake from your lungs to your bloodstream and help you recover faster.

If you test your progress by monitoring your heart rate, regular engagement in this type of training should result in your heart rate getting progressively lower each week as your fitness level increases. It's definitely a 'high five yourself' moment when this happens.

When building endurance, you'll want to focus on cardiovascular activities that increase your respiratory and heart rates. This includes exercise like walking or jogging, swimming, bike riding, and rope jumping. Keeping your heart, lungs, and circulatory system healthy will boost your overall fitness and increase your chances of ageing gracefully.

Resistance Training

Consider engaging in this type of training two to three times a week, with the length of your sessions being less critical than ensuring you exercise all the major muscle groups. Could you find an exercise that simultaneously uses them instead of isolating each muscle group? Also, posture is an overlooked but critical component of resistance training that will help reduce your injury chances.

Strength-based activities are often referred to as 'functional exercise', and trends, such as CrossFit, are mainly based on these movement patterns. If you are over 50, resistance training is vital for maintaining muscle mass and bone density and preventing falls. It's a good idea to use equipment, such as resistance bands, to reduce the risk of injury if you're just getting started; plus, they're portable and can easily be packed in a suitcase to use if you travel. No excuses!

What I love about resistance training is that we can integrate breathwork practice, balance, postural awareness, and power into this type of exercise. By staying mindful of how we integrate with this type of training, we engage our body and mind to cultivate a state of flow.

If you are under 30 years of age, it's super important to include resistance training as your bones develop towards their peak density. After this time, our bone density decreases yearly at a rate of approximately 1 percent for men and 2 to 4 percent for women. Resistance training can also assist in improving balance and muscle mass, both of which have a positive effect on decreasing the risk of developing osteoporosis.[19]

Seeking the advice of an exercise physiologist is a great place to start if you feel you have bodily limitations for optimal movement. Further, Pilates and yoga are easy ways to increase your strength without lifting weights. Both are excellent choices of activity to increase core strength to minimise back pain, postural issues, and incontinence. And they're fun!

Flexibility and Mobility Movements

Flexibility activities are essential for muscle balance, joint movement, and good posture and can prevent orthopaedic issues later in life. For example, tight hip muscles can cause wear to the cartilage, problems in the joint, and can impact other joints, such as your knees and ankles or even your neck. Gentle stretching and yoga are ideal choices to increase your mobility.

Starting your day with a short and straightforward stretching routine can reduce feelings of fatigue later in the day, so it's definitely worth the effort. I like to stretch in the kitchen while waiting for the kettle to boil.

Each muscle has a part called the Golgi tendon located near the junction of your tendon and muscle fibres. Its job is to protect your muscle from tearing by controlling the tension of a working muscle. Because of this, you'll want to hold each stretch for at least 30 seconds to allow the Golgi tendon to let the muscle relax enough to actually gain a little more length.

THE IDEAL COMBO FOR PAIN-FREE LIVING

Combining all types of training over a week is the most effective way to activate your body to reduce pain and improve your outcomes as you age. I'm all about being effective and efficient, so convergent activities, like circuit training, can save you time while helping you reach a place of optimum physical health. Some examples of combined training activities include swimming, cycling, jogging, or walking sessions for cardiovascular health, combined with regular weight training to target strength. Callisthenics and other bodyweight exercises, such as chin-ups or push-ups, are also excellent choices. Bodyweight activities can be performed anywhere because they rely on gravity, so you won't require weights. See – there's no excuse!

So many people need to remember flexibility. What's the point of being able to run fast and lift heavy objects if you can't touch your toes?

Enjoying stretches that focus on the chest and shoulder area, the back, knees and hips, hip flexors, gluteals, and hamstrings is essential for long-term mobility and will help you feel much better immediately.

"BUT I JUST WANT TO LOSE WEIGHT AND TONE UP!"

Trust me, I know the feeling, but you need to get fit to lose weight, tone up, and feel good. In the long run, merely changing your diet but not exercising can be detrimental to your future health. Unfortunately, a sedentary lifestyle can lead to losing muscle tissue and fluid, lulling you into the idea that you are successfully losing weight. It's all about body composition; that is, your ratio of bone to fat to muscle.

If you become fixated on weight loss and obsess over numbers on a set of scales, you may set yourself up for failure. By teaming healthy eating and excellent mindset practices with exercise, you're likely to lose fat, gain muscle, and potentially increase your bone density (that is, the weight of your skeleton). If this is the case, remember, a kilogram of muscle occupies less space than a kilogram of fat. This means that you may lose fat, gain muscle, and look trimmer, but the scales may not move – and that's still awesome.

WEIGHT LOSS VS. LIFE GAIN

Here's the thing about losing something… you generally find it again. And, nine out of ten times, you want to see it again. Think lost keys, mobile, your mojo, sleep (if only we could get that back). Yet, as a society, we obsess over 'losing weight'. And yes, you know where this is going – we generally find it again. Far too often, we regain more than we lost, which can be frustrating and not great for our mental health. Instead of focusing on losing weight, we should focus on all the things we gain when we make better choices about food and focus on our health and fitness, which generally results in weight loss.

What if we consider weight loss a by-product of life gain rather than the core goal?

Let's be honest, why do you want to lose weight? To rediscover your confidence? To gain energy? To keep up with your kids? To live longer? To find that mojo and achieve a healthier life?

Yes, yes, yes, yes, yes, and hell yes!

They're all things you want more of. And, when you make the right choices in pursuit of these goals, weight loss is a bonus. Winning!

If you're feeling less than fabulous and want to go from stuck to unstoppable, may I boldly suggest focusing on all the incredible things you will gain instead of what you want to lose? Should you commit to changing your lifestyle for the better?

Such a simple shift in mindset can make an incredible difference. So, what would you like more of in your life? It's a most excellent question.

Loz Lesson

To help you understand the benefits of each type of exercise and remember how often to undertake each one every week, download and print **Exercise Guide**. Pop it on your fridge or somewhere visually apparent around your home or office. You can do it! In fact, you have to. The end.

EXERCISE GUIDE
WHAT TO DO & HOW OFTEN

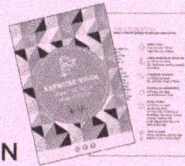

DOWNLOAD YOUR EXERCISE GUIDE **lozlife.com/book-exercise**

HOW MUCH EXERCISE WILL HELP YOU LOSE WEIGHT?

To lose weight, you need to balance your food intake with exercise. It's a simple mathematical equation. If you are ingesting more than you are burning off, you will put on weight. If you increase your training, burning off more energy than you put in, you will burn off body fat.

In its most basic form, the key to hitting your ideal weight is as simple as energy out exceeding energy in. Obviously, we want to consider what the 'energy in' is broken down to (in terms of macronutrient ratios, as covered in the Menu chapter). Still, if you consume more than you burn, that energy will need to be stored somewhere!

As a guideline, use the minimum daily requirement of 30 minutes of moderate exercise and double or even triple it, depending on how energetic you're feeling. At 30 minutes a day, you're protecting yourself against heart disease and other illnesses, and at 60 to 100 minutes, you'll be waving goodbye to those wobbly bits! See ya!

Ultimately, it does boil down to consistency so if you're not a regular exerciser, start small! People ask me, "What's the best workout I can do?", and my simple answer is always, "The one you will do!" If you can't commit to 30 minutes a day, try aiming for 10 minutes daily. Over a week, that's equivalent to 70 minutes of movement, which sure beats 30 minutes once a week.

I know so many people who make their whole journey about losing weight. Realistically, if you make it about feeling good and fitting into clothes more comfortably, you shift the goal to one that is far more meaningful and fulfilling, and you'll be setting yourself up for positive, healthy habits.

DEPRESSION

Did you know that more than one in five Australians suffer from mental illness, including anxiety and depression?[20] Fortunately, strength training and cardiovascular exercise are often successfully used as treatments. One trial found that exercise was as effective as some medications.[21] Research continues to confirm the connection between mental illness and the benefits of exercise. So, as you can see, it's not just about physical health; it's also about mental health, which is another reason to shake what your mumma gave you and get moving.

RECOVERING FROM INJURY

Most of us know someone who has sprained their ankle playing a sport, pulled a muscle running, or done their back gardening. If something like that has happened to you, you must gain advice from a health professional before you continue exercising.

If you have an injury, your treating medical professional will give you advice or a referral to a specialist or allied health professional. Medicare or private health insurance may partly cover appointments with a physiotherapist, occupational therapist, or exercise physiologist.

If you have already started your wellness journey, having to recover from injury can be disheartening and frustrating. Active injury prevention can help minimise the chances of hurting yourself in the first place.

It's a fact that most injuries occur from overuse of a joint or muscle or from simply going too hard, too fast, or too soon. It's surprisingly easy to do! It's recommended to start slowly and try out some fartlek training (yeah, it's a weird word) to make sure you don't overdo it at the beginning of your fitness program. A Swedish term for 'speed play', fartlek is when you alternate between a working period and an active rest period (for example, walk-run-walk-run). You might start with five minutes of walking and two minutes of running, gradually increasing the regimen each time you go out.

For the avid exerciser, a week off from exercising every 12 weeks will help prevent overuse injuries by allowing the soft tissues to recuperate. Alternatively, it's a good idea to alter your exercise routine every four to six weeks to challenge your body as your muscles get used to specific movement patterns. Mixing it up is a good thing.

Finding ways to incorporate incidental movement into everyday life is a great place to start if you're new to exercise. As a challenge for this week, try to devise ways to become more active each day. Maybe stand at your computer or go for a walk in the morning. Start small – ten minutes out of a whole day is perfect. It's a great start. You'll certainly feel better about it!

Loz Lesson

To help you track your daily movement activities, download and complete **You Can Do It!** and start working towards creating a new healthy habit over the next week and beyond.

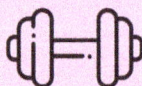

YOU CAN DO IT!
FITNESS TRACKER

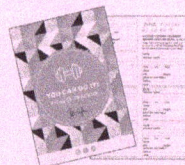

DOWNLOAD YOUR FITNESS TRACKER **lozlife.com/book-tracker**

The moral of the story? Move more! You can use daily activities to increase incidental movement and improve your health and fitness. It's really that simple. Walk more! Walk the dog, walk to work, walk to the shops. Always use the stairs over the escalator or lift, and park further from your destination and walk. Take a dance, aerobics, boxing, or yoga class, or join a sports team. Jump on the treadmill or bike at the gym. It all helps! Finally, when you are ready to take your health and fitness to the next level, consider hiring a coach or personal trainer to help you get safely and effectively started.

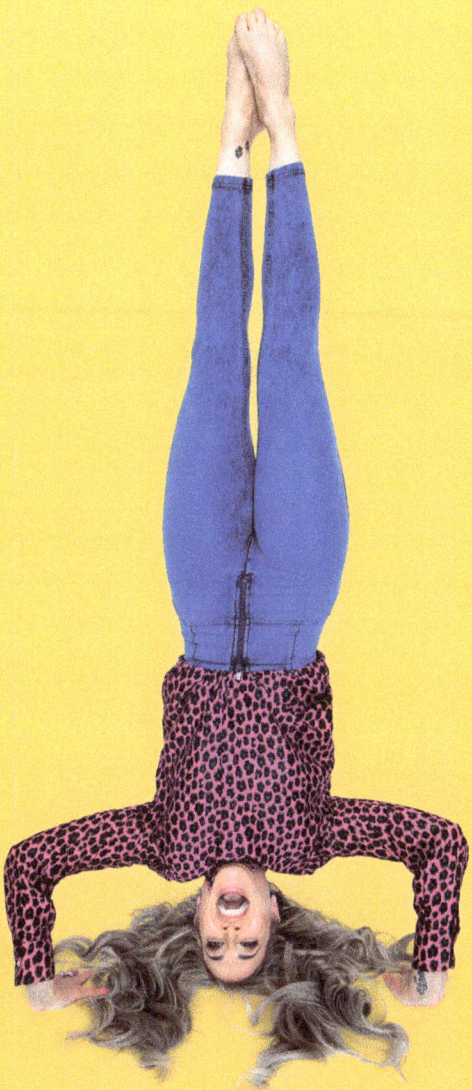
MASTERY

n this chapter, you will uncover the next step to creating a better you. The one that will truly transform your body, mind, and lifestyle... mastery. In fact, it used to be the last step in the Healthy Habit Hierarchy before I added the all-vital chapter on Mentorship. More on that later.

Simply put, this is a place in your lifelong journey where you keep doing all the things I have taught you throughout this book and teach others to do the same. This chapter will give you the tools to live and grow with integrity, authenticity, and passion.

Repetition is the absolute key to mastery and the source of skill. Mastery is simply about understanding something, feeling it, and doing it instinctively. There is a powerful driving force inside every human being that, once unleashed, can make any vision, dream, or desire a reality.

The path we take towards mastering anything – our careers, finances, relationships – comes down to three simple steps: modelling, immersion, and repetition. Friends, that is mastery.

It's time to trade expectations for the appreciation of the life you are blessed to live. Imagine how incredible it would feel to consistently live a pain-free life where you could kick arse at everything you choose to pursue. F*ck yes!

For long-term, sustainable results, we must be able to adapt to new environments, new information, and new circumstances. We need to move beyond the necessary steps of taking action as a knee-jerk response. Proactivity developing a core personal health philosophy and creating an environment that heals and nurtures are key to lifelong vitality.

Achievement is a science, but fulfilment... well, that's an art! You have the choice to design an enriching life that you love. The power is literally in your hands, my friend.

Success is simple. Do what's right, the right way, at the right time, and magic will happen. There's a suitable time for everything. Everything always happens at the right time. Sometimes you have to make something happen by planning, goal setting, and taking action. Other times you have to wait for it. If things don't go the way you planned, it just wasn't meant to be. Sometimes that's hard to manage, but it's the truth. The trick is to be persistent and patient and surrender to a universal force far more significant than you. Surrendering isn't always easy.

Trust the timing of your life because it will be perfect. Nothing is ever in the way. It's just on the way to something more empowering, gratifying, and fulfilling. Funnily enough, life's roughest storms prove the strength of our anchors. I love that analogy. A smooth sea never made a skilled sailor. Remember, we can't control the winds, but we can adjust our sails.

While I'm trotting out the great boating-related quotes… a ship in the harbour is safe, but that is not what ships are built for. Nuff said.

Let's get deep. The world's best and most beautiful things cannot be seen or even touched. They must be felt with the heart. Beauty comes from loving yourself. If you had told me ten years ago that I could love myself in all my authentic fullness, the good and the weird, I would have told you to bugger off!

On my mastery journey, I have not so accidentally fallen in love with my unstoppable life and the discipline it takes to perpetuate it. I love my freedom of speech and how my eyes get dark when I'm tired because my physical and emotional selves are so deeply connected. I love that I have learnt to trust people with my heart, even if it means it may get broken. I am proud of everything that I am and will become. I hope, one day soon, you can say the same.

BECOME A HEALTHY HABIT MASTER

We are creatures of habit, which can be a good thing if our habits are healthy.

Learning a new habit can be the saviour of our future selves. Uncovering new patterns can release us from lousy past behaviours and stop us from being tainted by our past mistakes, failures, and setbacks… the things that we've allowed to haunt us for years.

A word here about the concept of success – too many people confuse success with money and fame. In isolation, these tangible outcomes are not 'success' and, on their own, cannot sustainably bring fulfilment. When you think about it, success without fulfilment is the ultimate failure. It's all a bit cliché, but real progress is about chasing the intangibles: the journey, the experience, and the feeling mastery brings. Not the cold, hard cash and fancy cars.

No one ever became a success by chance. Mastery, and the achievements that come with it, are about taking chances by just doing. There's no time like now to allow yourself the opportunity to add up a stack of tiny changes and formulate a lifetime of healthy habits from here on in.

We can all relate to the concept of the honeymoon period: that fresh new time when you start something new, like a relationship or a self-improvement program, and your enthusiasm is super high. The momentum motivates you. You are driven and drawn to the goal by the pleasure of what you want or are pulled and propelled away from the pain of what you don't want. The problem is that we live in an age of continuous, unrelenting change, and unfortunately motivation diminishes with time. When inspiration leaves you, you need willpower. No one has an endless supply of willpower. Willpower dwindles whenever you persuade yourself to do something you don't want to do. So, when your will has decreased enough, temptation slips in – and temptation is an arsehole. The thing about temptation is that it further depletes willpower, and then you find yourself with no will by the end of the day. This is precisely why most people find it hard by the evening to stick to a diet after eating healthy all day long.

So, momentum, menu, mindset, and movement are good. But if the connection between mastery and momentum is missing in the cycle, you may find yourself drifting off course with speed, only to get stuck again. It's a shitty, vicious cycle to get stuck in. The trick is to build strong, foundational, lifelong resilience to help you handle life's ebbs and flows and unlock and unleash abundance, fulfilment, joy, and, ultimately, success.

Do you think about how to brush your teeth or how to drive your car? Nope. You just do it. It has been suggested that our subconscious dictates 95 per cent of our lives, putting us on autopilot for the everyday things we have already taught our unconscious mind to do. This is habit-forming stuff, people. We can consciously choose to create new pathways to form healthy habits. Through practise, these become established patterns of behaviour and actions over time, and we won't need as much motivation and willpower to keep doing them. Get my drift? Then you are winning at life!

So, let's start putting together a plan to create that new pathway to a healthy habit.

PREPARE AND MEASURE CONVENIENTLY

I spoke earlier about the importance of measuring success using the SMART acronym. If you've forgotten, go back to the Mindset chapter and refresh your memory. I'll wait here…

If you are about to start a movement habit, prepare yourself so you have what you need to get it done. A pair of comfortable shoes come to mind if you are going to walk. Who doesn't feel inspired by new activewear? An electronic activity monitor will help you measure your steps towards creating a healthy habit. Fact: statistically, the act of measuring your daily efforts with a device will lead you to walk 27 percent more than those who don't use one.[22]

It's all about putting in a little bit of preparation to make activities convenient and easy, so pop those running shoes by the front door where you can see them. I believe it's crucial to be on your A game when it comes to preparation, just in case your willpower is a little down. Nothing is more frustrating than not achieving your goals on time because you were underprepared. Eliminate that excuse today.

REPEAT AND TRACK

In previous chapters, I let you know about my Post-it note system, my success list, and journalling strategies to track where I am going. I also love to use apps and good old-fashioned calendars to keep tabs on my habits. No matter which one resonates with you, after using the same technique for more than four weeks, you will find it is habitual and something you hardly even think about doing.

Stats show that you need to repeat patterns of behaviour for 66 days to form a habit.[23] That's essentially nine-and-a-bit weeks, so four weeks is just under halfway! You can do it. Try using a planner or a diary to plot your success strategy if that suits your lifestyle better. Remember, repetition is the key to results.

Loz Lesson

To help you plan your success, download
66-Day Tracker and complete it daily
to steer you towards your path to mastery

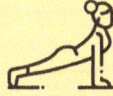

66 DAY TRACKER
TO MASTERY

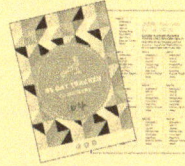

DOWNLOAD YOUR 66 DAY TRACKER **lozlife.com/book-66-tracker**

DON'T FORGET TO ADD FUN

If you need someone to get you through, reach out to a partner and make it fun. Having your partner, best friend, or other support person join you on your path to success makes it doubly rewarding and way more fun.

You don't have to go it alone!

HANG AROUND PEOPLE WHO INSPIRE YOU

Spending time in the company of people who inspire you to strive for excellence is a sure-fire way to help keep the momentum burning. Motivational speaker, Jim Rohn, is said to have coined the phrase, "You're the average of the five people you spend the most time with." This means that we are all influenced by our friends, so it's a good idea to have a close inner circle of positive and supportive people, some of whom are further along the path to where we want to be, to raise our average.

I don't know about you, but I love being around successful people! It's addictive and oh-so-inspiring.

By frequently using these habitual steps, you are creating a new pathway. Once formed, you can move on to the next habit as you break down those goals into measurable milestones.

SPREAD THE LOVE AND PAY IT FORWARD

Go on and smile today… it might just be the key that fits the lock to someone's heart. A cute thought, right? Life is effortless, but most insist on making it highly complicated! Sometimes life can be challenging. This is a given. But never forget that you, yes YOU, *do* make a difference. Whatever it is that you are doing will be worthwhile. You are loved, and just a simple smile today may bring hope to the life of another, even if that person is you. You don't need to be a superhero to make someone's day better by being a part of it, but you might feel like one. Cape is not required. Kindness is being someone's reason to smile. Look for opportunities, lead by example, and be the change. Helping someone else realise the possibilities of their wildest dreams through loving kindness is the ultimate secret to mastery.

Secret – the more positive energy you give out, freely and without expectations, the more you'll receive back in spades.

Remember from a few chapters back: voluntary simplicity can be considered the ultimate form of sophistication. Always keep in mind the KISS (keep it simple, stupid) principle, which can be more challenging than it seems, but sometimes you have to work hard initially to simplify your life. Honestly, it's worth it in the end because once you get there, you can move mountains! Collect the tiny yet beautiful moments that today offers you because one day, down the track, you may look back and realise how big those little pieces of your life were. The small moments really do matter.

If it's not making me money, better, or happy, then realistically I don't have time for it. Lately, I've been putting pen to paper, my money where my mouth is, and my heart on my sleeve. These actions make me realise that I am designed with an unstoppable spirit. You might be a work in progress, but every day you're getting a little wiser, a bit better, and a whole lot stronger.

Real beauty? It only begins when you decide to be yourself, let go of the past, and move forward with integrity and grace. It's taken me years to realise my real strength as a woman and a human being. I've learnt that real power comes from within. No amount of physical strength can match authentic inner prowess (although muscles *are* cute!). My inner sass is strong… but so is my body.

Life… wasn't meant to be easy, by any means, but what of that anyway? We must all discover perseverance, resilience, and confidence in ourselves. We must believe we are gifted at something, and that one thing, whatever it may be, at whatever cost, must be attained. Live your life with your highest values at the forefront of every moment. It's your choice to go into every single day and find that inner strength behind your innate beauty so the world will not blow out your candle.

These days, glitter is my favourite colour, and I spread it everywhere (and don't you dare try to tell me that glitter isn't a colour!). Nothing can dim the light that shines from within, so why be afraid to sparkle? I believe that a compassionate heart radiates rays of beauty that remove the clouds of self-doubt. Each time a person passes by you and you say hello, imagine you're igniting that person's internal candle. The more positivity, love, and light you reflect, the more light is mirrored your way. Sharing beautiful hellos with your voice, or the silence of a smile, is the quickest way to earn spiritual brownie points. You should start seeing hellos as minor declarations of grace and gratitude. Every time you say hello to a stranger, your heart acknowledges that we are all family and in this magnificent life journey together. We are all just walking each other home. May your soul radiate light and love, and you leave a sprinkle of magic wherever you go!

The art of mastering deep fulfilment can sometimes be a challenge, but it's all about practise, and it's always worth the effort.

Loz Lesson

For your next exercise, download and complete **Identify Your Hidden Strengths** to pinpoint the critical areas that give you a sense of meaning and purpose. You never know; you may come across some patterns in your strengths and uncover a new way to help add value to the lives of others as you travel on your Mastery journey.

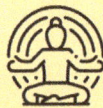

IDENTIFY YOUR HIDDEN STRENGTHS

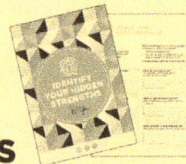

DOWNLOAD YOUR ID YOUR HIDDEN STRENGTHS **lozlife.com/book-strengths**

CLIENT STORY
– FINDING THE PATH TO MASTERY

I'm not going to lie – mastery takes discipline. Even so, that doesn't mean we must sacrifice *all* the things we enjoy, even if they aren't technically 'good' for us. Often, we can find a middle ground.

Caroline and Peter ran a busy electrical business with a large cohort of contractors under their supervision. Although working together proved challenging, it was also very rewarding because they could share their successes on their journey. Their kids had grown up and left home, so, as empty nesters, they found time each evening to wind down over a 'glass' of wine. Unfortunately, this glass turned into several bottles each night, plus the excessive cheese and crackers that went down nicely with a drop of red. Both Caroline and Peter had gained weight, and they had stopped playing social sports because they were always too tired.

The couple brought me into their workplace to help their team improve their performance. They had experienced a high level of absenteeism and wanted to invest in their team to help them develop better habits for more productivity.

Now, I'm a believer that the habits of the business owners and leadership team will always funnel down into the team culture. As Caroline and Peter's lifestyle habits started to slip, there was a direct correlation to their team morale shifting.

Over ten weeks, the team, including the owners, undertook my Boss Loz Healthy Habit Overhaul program. Under my guidance and supervision, participants are encouraged to develop new healthy habits and be accountable to a support buddy to ensure they stick to their goals. With weekly team calls and homework, this immersive program is full-on but yields incredibly transformative results for those who follow the process and do the work. Every participant's outcomes are different but intricately tied to their values and lifestyle goals, following the blueprint of my Healthy Habit Hierarchy (the six M's).

It was super important for Caroline and Peter to still be able to enjoy an alcoholic beverage but within their scope of control and as a conduit for downtime in which a deeper connection would be anchored, rather than escapism and habit. At the end of the program, not only were the couple able to enjoy wine in moderation, but they went back to playing touch and netball, lost a few kilos of body fat, and found better self-governance to regulate their habits to match the lifestyle they truly craved – and their team reaped the benefits of a new, health-centric culture, where everyone could thrive.

INVEST IN A COACH OR MENTOR

What a great segue into the next chapter – my new addition to my Healthy Habit Hierarchy. In so many beautiful ways, coaching is an excellent tool to help you accelerate progress by providing greater focus and awareness of choice. By aligning yourself with someone with experience in the areas you want to master, a mentor can provide you with a path to model because success leaves clues.

Either way, you can gain insight into the strategies and techniques others have used… learn from their successes and failures because both are teaching moments. This will allow you to bypass unnecessary roadblocks more swiftly and arrive at your goals faster. Coaching and mentoring will help you concentrate on where you are now, what you need to do, and where you want to be. Overall, a powerful self-development strategy and investment in yourself leads to change and tangible results.

Time and again, people supported by a wellness or life coach measurably improve their mental, physical, and spiritual health for long-term results. It's about following a structured plan and taking small steps towards healthier behaviours. Coaching essentially helps us stay accountable while we create sustainable changes to our lifestyle through habit alteration. As a coach, I help people play in a space beyond their perceived capabilities, helping them realise they can achieve anything (within reason, of course). Oh, and I freaking love coaching and mentorship.

Ultimately, coaching encourages self-reliance, life satisfaction, planning skills, and efficiency in both the workplace and the home. It also provides practical communication skills to transfer to other parts of your life.

More on coaching and mentorship soon...

As you have learnt from this chapter, while it's essential to always celebrate your accomplishments, it's equally imperative to raise the bar a little bit each time you succeed. We all deserve love and affection, including our own.

It's super important to remember that only you have control over the way your life feels. In the end, mastery is all about making it your life's work to keep evolving, growing, and strengthening your individual and collaborative development with your community to become a kick-arse human being. Even if you stumble, keep moving forward, because you have got this! Simple, hey? Oh... and you're never alone. Ever.

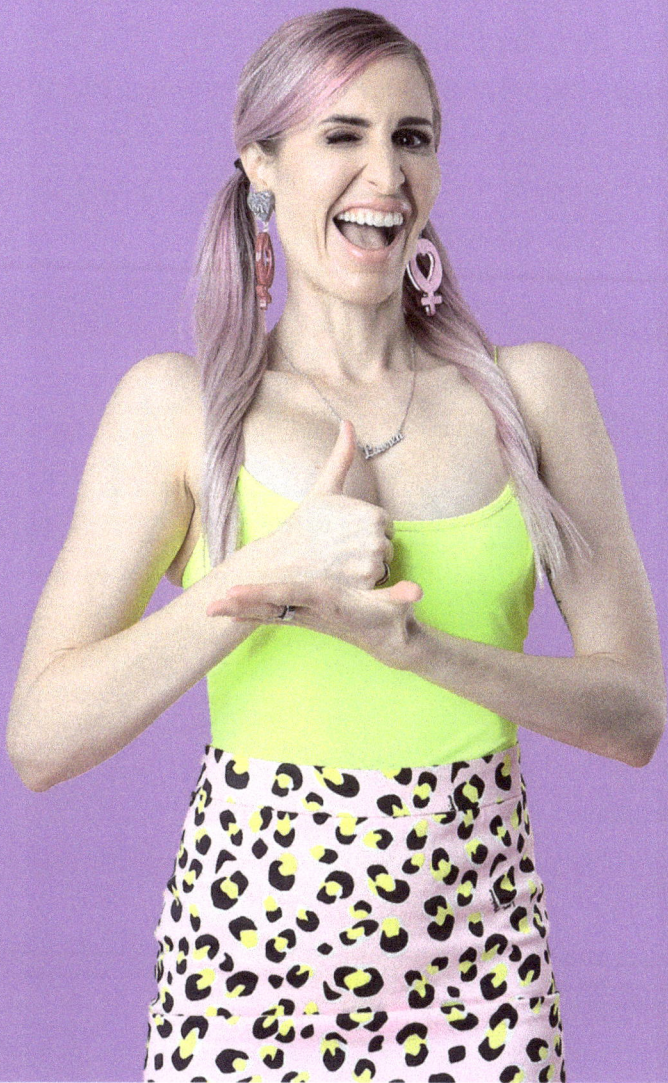
MENTORSHIP

"Steve, thank you for being a mentor and a friend. Thanks for showing that what you build can change the world. I will miss you." Mark Zuckerberg, Facebook CEO, tweets about his mentor, Steve Jobs, the former Apple CEO.[24]

In this final chapter, we dive deep into the mentoring world. What is it, who does it, and why do you need it?

Cultures live, prosper, and die from the leadership and contributions of those who actively engage in that culture. Leading by example is the essence of being a great leader and empowering others to level up their lives.

Mentoring is about helping someone who may be at the start of their journey and facilitating the achievement of their dreams so they can kick goals, which you do by sharing your expertise and experience. A great mentor is someone willing to help and provide guidance while still being open to learning from *their* mentors. You can be both a mentor and a mentee at the same time, or even a co-mentor, where you and someone at a similar stage will mentor each other. A true mentor is someone who has reached a certain level of success in their life or career and wants to share that knowledge to help others. Advisors, consultants, and coaches can be great mentors, but a great mentor doesn't have to be any of those things. Just because you're a coach doesn't make you a mentor.

At the end of the chapter, head to lozlife.com for some exercises designed to help you find your perfect mentor!

Love him or hate him, even social media megabucks guru, Mark Zuckerberg, has benefited from being mentored (by none other than Steve Jobs, the former CEO of Apple) to help him along the way. I'm not suggesting you start frantically emailing the CEOs of global companies and begging them to become your mentor. I recommend you get serious about finding a mentor who can help you take your life, career, and passions to the next level.

Mentoring isn't new. In fact, it's been helping transform people's lives for thousands of years. There was a character in mythology called Mentor, entrusted to care for Odysseus's son while Odysseus headed off to fight in the Trojan War. Yep, that's how far back mentoring goes. It's possible that even cavepeople mentored each other in fire lighting and mammoth hunting.

These days, more than 70 percent of Fortune 500 companies run formal mentoring programs.[25] In case you don't know what a Fortune 500 company is, it's one of the 500 largest US companies, making serious bank. Big cashola. They're a big deal. If they think mentoring is a promising idea, then it's probably something to consider.

So, let's look at what makes a great mentor, how you can find the right one, and how it can help to transform your life.

WHAT IS A MENTOR? AND WHAT MAKES A 'GREAT' MENTOR?

In its simplest terms, a mentor is someone who has reached a certain level of professional experience on their journey and is at a stage where they want to give back. Mentorship is a way of helping to inspire others through conscious leadership to help them on their journey. But a great mentor is somebody willing to help and provide guidance while still opening themselves up to learning from their mentors.

True mentors lead lives of their own design and want to share their knowledge to help others. By sharing their experiences, mentors can help their mentees 'unlock' something in themselves.

It's a conscious decision to become a *mentor.*

Find the person already succeeding at what you want to do. It could be business, life, goals, passions – anything. As long as they're further along the road on the journey than you and achieving the goals you want to achieve one day, they're potentially great mentors.

SO, IS MENTORING JUST ABOUT BUSINESS AND CAREER GROWTH?

Mentoring is absolutely not just about business and career growth. In fact, we've all had mentors around us our entire lives – our parents, family, teachers, and friends. They've all been our mentors since the day we were born.

We might seek mentors for a range of unique needs and desires, from wanting to transition into a leadership position, improving our health and vitality, learning how to connect with a professional network – the list is endless.

Generally, we seek out a mentor when we realise that we have an end goal, but we don't quite know how to get there. A mentor can provide a new perspective that can make a difference in a mentee's life. They should be able to recommend tasks, provide resources if necessary, and help you develop steps of action to get you closer to your goal. Excellent mentoring is about helping the mentee do things correctly and ensuring they feel confident when doing them.

For example, suppose a mentor is helping a mentee to become better at networking. In that case, they help facilitate conversations or accompany the mentee to networking events and encourage them to observe them networking.

That role modelling is a terrific way for us to learn, sort of a 'monkey see, monkey do' scenario. It's how we learn as we grow up and how the animal kingdom passes on its knowledge to the next generation.

CAN A MENTOR ALSO BE A ROLE MODEL?

A mentor can be a role model, someone you admire, or someone who's achieved what you want. A professional mentor-mentee relationship is usually formalised, but anybody can be a mentor. It's just how you frame it.

If you use the example of your mother – usually your first mentor – she helps you to grow, teaches you how to solve problems, and provides solutions and frameworks for you as you grow up. Really, a professional mentor is not that dissimilar.

Whether you agree to a formal, paid, or unpaid mentorship, a mentor is there to help you develop and grow. A great mentor will stimulate your thinking and help you see outside the box. But keep in mind that not all mentors and mentees are going to be a great fit. You need to find the right fit, just like the perfect pair of jeans.

You need to feel comfortable, and a great mentor – or pair of jeans – will help you feel more confident and ready to conquer the world.

GOOD MENTORS HELP FOSTER INDEPENDENCE – THEY DON'T DO IT FOR YOU!

For mentees, just remember, your mentor isn't there to hold your hand (or wipe your bum). They're there to teach you how to achieve, grow, develop, and thrive independently. They're not going to do it for you. Instead, they'll give you the road map to take you where you want to go, and then it's up to you.

For mentors, remember that the end goal is to teach your mentee to do it for themselves. You don't want to do it for them. And, while you might have to be a bit more hands-on at the start of the relationship, make sure you slowly step back as your mentee develops their confidence and starts to lean into the person they want to become.

The mentor-mentee relationship should include a deep level of trust, respect, and confidence, but, like a small bird with a broken wing that you've nursed back to health, at some stage, you need to know when to set them free and let them fly solo.

SHOULD MENTORS AND MENTEES BE FRIENDS?

Whether mentors and mentees should be friends depends on the level of the relationship. 'Friends' probably isn't the right word for a mentor-mentee relationship, but you will naturally become well acquainted with one another during your connection. You're building a level of rapport that can grow into friendship, but make sure, if you develop a friendship, it doesn't disrupt the boundaries and dynamics of your professional association.

One of the problems with becoming friends with your mentor or mentee is that, as a consequence, the expectations on both sides can be skewed.

I've had lots of friends that have come to me as clients in a professional setting, but then they'd have an expectation that they'd get a hefty discount. So, the challenge is that you might be happy to give your family and friends a special rate for whatever service or products you provide as part of your professional life but, remember, if people invest in a service or a product, they're going to have a lot more respect for it than if you make it too cheap.

If you're a mentee and you're not paying your mentor, maybe you can give your mentor a discount on your services or products to thank them, but neither side should ever expect it.

NETWORKING TO FIND YOUR MENTOR

Let's be brutally honest here: for many of us, going to a networking event and being stuck in a room full of professional people can be like the ninth circle of hell. It's scary. You're putting yourself out there, which can be confronting, and not everyone has the gift of the gab when it comes to selling themselves to strangers.

If you know who's likely to be attending the networking event, get busy on LinkedIn and learn everything you can about them. Who on that guest list could be your ideal mentor?

Striking up a conversation in a roomful of successful-looking people can be challenging, but, like anything, it's a muscle you must develop. Toughen up, kid! Practise in front of the mirror. Have some opening conversational gambits, arm yourself with your business cards, wear an outfit that makes you feel great, and then force yourself in.

Remember why you're doing it in the first place. Think about your goal and what you want to achieve. Then go get 'em, tiger! You got this.

Think of a mentor as a source of inspiration who will help, advise, guide, and coach you along the way.

SHOULD MENTORS AND MENTEES SET BOUNDARIES?

As a mentor, you'll need to set some boundaries around how and when you're available and ensure you're clear about your expectations regarding the relationship. I recommend you do it from the get-go. A mentor needs to be really available and responsive because that's what you're there for – to be open to offering support, advice, and help. BUT, and it's a big but, you need to ensure your mentee knows how and when they can get in touch.

There's no point in becoming a mentor if you have no space for people. The expectation in that relationship dynamic is that you are available to be called upon when somebody has an issue. What you need to clarify from the very start of the relationship is your preferred channels of communication and how frequently you're able to respond.

So, being clear about what that communication looks like is a critical task for both the mentor and the mentee. I know, in my own journey, I've had many issues with people overstepping communication boundaries because I haven't really been enforcing them. I hadn't set the expectation clearly.

I have a policy where mentees can ask me a question or tell me what's happening with them any time they want but with the clear understanding that I'll only respond at certain times. That way, the mentee can contact me at any time that's convenient, but they know they won't get an immediate response. I also request that they ask questions in dot points to make it easier – don't send me a giant novel via email – and I ask that they try to limit emails to once per week. Email is a much better way to communicate; people put more thought into what they want to say. Avoid leaving unprepared or jumbled messages on voicemail that the mentor has to decipher.

When you're mentoring other people, if you're filling from an empty cup because you're constantly at the mercy of people texting at 2 am, which has happened to me in the past, how can you expect to show up for that person and really honour what it is you're expected to bring to that relationship?

You've also got to be really good at respecting confidentiality because what happens in a mentoring session stays in a mentoring session. When you develop that depth of relationship with somebody in a mentoring capacity, your mentee will want to share, and they should feel safe to do that.

As a mentor, it's essential to develop your own network and surround yourself with other people because you can't be everything to everyone. For example, suppose you have a mentee who asks a question you can't answer. Rather than giving an answer that's outside your scope or, worse, making it up, you can refer them to somebody in your trusted partnership network who could answer with more detail and accuracy.

BEING A GOOD MENTEE

A good mentee does the work. They complete any tasks their mentor sets, and they take them seriously.

Here's a good example – imagine you're going to a physiotherapist for a sore back. The physio will give you a series of exercises to do at home, which will help you recover. What happens if you don't do the exercises? You don't get the value out of seeing your physio; your back doesn't get any better, and you're wasting your time and theirs.

So, in a nutshell, my advice is this – do the f*cking work, get down, and be responsible.

Value your mentor's time by being available and communicating openly and clearly.

If your expectation is that your mentor is going to be available to you, you need to be available for them. Make sure you keep your channels of communication open for that person.

With my own mentor, for example, I always pick up if he calls me, even if I'm with a client. I'll just excuse myself to the client, call him back, and let him know I'm with a client. The reason I do that? Because I want to make it clear that I value his time.

It can be as simple as, "Hey, mate, I'm just with a client. Can I please call you back?"

Very occasionally, if I can't get to my phone, I will let it go to the message bank, but then I'll send a quick text to say I'm with the client. It's about making sure that your communication is a two-way street. You can't just expect to be communicated to and then not communicate back.

DO I PAY MY MENTOR?

Some mentors are paid, and others do it as an unpaid service. It depends on the relationship's dynamic and what you agree to early on. A mentor will be there to help support somebody on their way. They also act in the role of advisor when required.

Mentors who act as consultants for you may expect to be paid, so make sure you have your relationship parameters clearly defined before you kick off.

STAKE IT TILL YOU MAKE IT

You must have skin in the game even if you don't technically 'pay' your mentor. If you're somebody seeking personal development through modelling and mentorship, think about what will make you show up and do the work.

People don't value time as much as they love money. People with money at stake are likelier to show up and be more honest.

Here's an example: I'm in a mastermind, which is a form of mentorship and peer support, and I pay a subscription fee to be part of it. Now, it's a relatively small investment but I know that if I'm going to spend X number of dollars a month, I will get out of bed and hop on a Zoom call every week at 6:30 am to show up for these people.

BE WILLING TO DO THE WORK (INCLUDING YOUR HOMEWORK!)

First, make sure your mentor is a good fit by using helpful tools such as DiSC personality profiling, which can help determine if your mentor is the right one for you. Make sure you are both on the same page regarding goals and what you want to achieve.

The right mentor for you should be good at understanding and articulating your goals, but, before they can do that, *you* need to know your plans. You need to be able to communicate clearly, be authentic, and learn to express what it is you really want. Just remember, if you can't share your goals, how the hell will a stranger be able to do it? And then, will you get the help and advice you truly need? Nope.

Don't be afraid to talk openly about your expectations and aspirations; don't be frightened or embarrassed to share some audacious goals. While they might not seem to be in the realm of possibility in the early stages, let your mentor know that you're not afraid to think big. Because the bolder you are and the more you share your wildest ambitions, the better your mentor will understand what you want to achieve.

When you communicate openly and clearly with your mentor, they'll be able to teach you in a way that fits your learning style, whether, for example, that means talking a problem out with somebody or drawing it – whatever works best for you.

And, finally, do the work. Show up and *do the work*. Show your mentor that you value their time and expertise and respect their knowledge and experience. If they set you a task, ensure you do it on time and make it the best work you can do. Otherwise, you're just wasting their time and yours.

SHOULD MENTORING SESSIONS BE FORMAL?

Mentoring sessions should have a certain amount of formality and preparation to ensure that both the mentor and the mentee feel the session has some value. Mentees should always come to meetings with their mentors armed with an agenda. Don't just rock up as if you have a casual catch-up with a friend. Know what you want to talk about, be clear on what areas you need their help with, and be prepared. It's up to the mentee, not the mentor, to prepare for these sessions. You must go in with a clear idea of what you want to achieve from the session. Your mentor will have little feedback or advice if you can't articulate your purpose or goals.

Be responsible for your own learning and if your mentor gives you a task, keep in mind that it's there for your own benefit. Again, and I can't stress this enough, do the f*cking work. Take responsibility. Put the time in so when you meet up, there's something to talk about, and they can then give you feedback. Read books, educate yourself, listen to podcasts, read blogs, read articles, go to events, and do things you need to do that will help you show up for that mentor. Get on point.

The other side of that coin is that your mentor might say constructively critical things about you. Understand that it's feedback, not failure, so don't start feeling defensive if your mentor gives you constructive criticism or feedback. Remember that your mentor is there to help you, and constructive criticism is designed to help you improve, grow, develop, and learn.

TRUST THE PROCESS

Developing a profound sense of trust is at the core of a mentor-mentee relationship. Use that wisely. Don't abuse trust; if there are boundaries, don't cross them. Just remember that your mentor is engaged as your trusted advisor.

Having a mentor shouldn't feel like a chore; the relationship you develop, the advice you receive, and the tasks you're given should all feel engaging, fun, fruitful, and joyous. You should feel like you're getting something out of it. If it feels like a chore, then chances are you're paired up with the wrong mentor.

CLIENT STORY
– MENTORS MAKE A DIFFERENCE

As a mentee, I have experienced the value a great mentor can provide, and, over the years, I have extended the same support to others.

Tom had been a PT for a few years now but was tired of his clients only getting suboptimal results and then leaving him. He was motivated and didn't mind working long hours, but he was starting to

Remember that if you are not paying your mentor, they're doing this for you *as a gift.*

burn out. Tom struggled with sales and hated pitching himself on social media – he would rather be in the gym helping people. With living costs soaring, he was finding that many clients were unable to budget for PT sessions, so he knew he needed to find another way to keep his business buoyant.

Tom and I connected in a fitness professionals group on Facebook. He really liked my approach to habit change and how I integrated movement into a much bigger puzzle. As a PT, Tom's scope of practice was actually quite limited, and it was really challenging for him to deliver the types of results he knew he could without stepping outside his legal scope. What Tom didn't realise was that about 60 percent of personal trainers leave the industry within the first six months of their careers due to the very same challenges he was experiencing. Sales felt 'icky'. Invoicing and admin took up heaps of his time. He was literally just exchanging time for money and then had no time left to enjoy the fruits of his labours because he was exhausted.

I invited Tom to complete my Healthy Habit Hierarchy Academy (H3A) upskills program: Healthy Habit Fundamentals. I knew that the key skills he would develop from my syllabus would bridge his knowledge gaps and give him the confidence to help his clients with not only their movement but also their momentum, menu, and mindset so they could develop their own self-mastery and he could then really help them skyrocket their success.

Upon completing his Loz Life training, Tom really wanted to continue his personal development. We formalised a mentorship agreement, and I brought Tom on as a Loz Life coach, where he would receive ongoing support from me and my team. Through conscious connection with other high achievers who are on a mission to help others live unstoppable lives, Tom has really up-levelled his circle of support, positively impacting his coaching business. He has now created a business where he and his clients can both thrive. By creating a better strategy that aligns with his long-term lifestyle goal, he continues to receive mentorship from me, as needed.

TAKING IT TO THE NEXT LEVEL – BEYOND MENTORING

The next step beyond the mentor-mentee relationship is a mastermind, another version of mentorship based on peer-level support.

Think of it as a co-facilitation process where you've got a facilitator who's not necessarily an expert but someone who has an interest in a particular area. The facilitator will bring together people with similar goals, ideas, ideologies, and belief systems who are looking to improve some specific area of their lives.

A mastermind allows you to express what you're going through and what challenges you're facing, then enabling you to brainstorm with your peers. During a session, everybody gets some time in the hot seat. It's like a peer-supported mentorship, where you're all each other's mentors and mentees.

For example, in my mastermind group, we have an ENT surgeon in the States who is super good at what she does, but she's looking to improve areas of her personal health. So, in that capacity, I can advise on certain things and give some evidence on health and fitness. At the same time, she's an incredibly skilled human so if I needed to learn something about her speciality, she'd be there to offer me help and advice. Basically, we're both the mentors and the mentees in that situation. It's about sharing our expertise with our peers.

Being a mentor means helping to inspire confidence in others and encouraging independence to help people follow their purpose and achieve their goals. It's about prepping others to go and actively seek challenges that will get them to where they want to be.

As Dr John Demartini says, "Maximum performance and maximum achievements occur at the border of support and challenge."[26] So, when you're challenged by something, when something's hard and you seek the proper help, for example, through a mentor, that's when you grow the most and perform at your best.

When stuff gets hard, you (wo)man up and keep going. Find your network, do the work, show up, have some skin in the game, and never give up!

MORE ON MASTERMINDS

"It is wise to surround yourself with people who are consciously expanded, clear about their mission, inspired by what they are doing, and who would love to see you achieve your objectives and dreams because they also want to achieve, and they know if they help others achieve, they help themselves in turn to the same."[27]

– Dr John Demartini

They say a rising tide lifts all ships, which is precisely why having an exceptional circle of influence is vital to your success. Managing your circle is not only about your existing relationships but also about enhancing your connections by attracting the type of people you'd like to hang around in five to ten years. This is where masterminds can be a powerful tool to supercharge your network.

The concept of a mastermind has been around for donkey's years. Does 'Knights of the Round Table' sound familiar? That, my friends, is an excellent example of a peer-supported network of like-minded individuals coming together over shared values to help each other meet a common goal through accountability – that is, a mastermind.

In these small groups, the collective usually meets regularly to brainstorm, solve problems, dissect challenges, and support other masterminders by providing a safe space to discuss anything within the group scope. A nominated party facilitates the conversation, and an agenda is typically set to keep sessions flowing.

Now, this sounds like mentoring, right? Well, masterminds are similar, but there are some distinct differences between the two:

* Masterminds are groups of people. Mentoring is a one-on-one relationship.

* Masterminds are about an equal flow of giving and receiving support and advice. Mentorship is usually more about receiving help.

* Masterminds follow a structured frequency – usually weekly, fortnightly, monthly, or quarterly. With a mentor, there's more flexibility with your engagement schedule.

Masterminds have provided tremendous opportunities to connect with like-minded individuals who are equally as driven and energised as I am. These connections have been invaluable, and peer-supported accountability has kept my momentum gliding along at a rapid but manageable pace for maximum impact on my goals. Remember, anyone who's successful hasn't gotten there on their own.

The benefits of belonging to a mastermind are broad, but, from personal experience, here's what I've found most impactful about hanging out regularly with a bunch of awesome folks:

1. **Speedy access to support when you need it** – Masterminds are a place where you can speak the truth and expect to receive it in return, so when you need a community to help you navigate obstacles and celebrate success, your group will always be there to encourage you to be your best self.

2. **The ability to create an incredible network** – Not only can peer support keep you focused and energised, but sharing contacts and connections outside the group is a great way to build trusted introductions to more aligned people.

3. **Skill enhancement** – Because everyone in the group is at a different point on their journey and can offer vast skills, experience, strengths, and weaknesses, you'll find that, as a collective, you'll complement each other to further elevate individual skills and your perception of success.

4. **Creation and sharing of ideas** – I like to consider masterminds 'think tanks', as they're like little idea incubators where you can gain outside perspectives and feedback from people you trust.

Many of my mentors have become my mastermind peers, and I now find myself levelling up my circle of influence quite rapidly. It's all about the power of proximity. I like to keep a list of my most impactful connections and ensure I connect with these people regularly, even if it's just a simple text message to drop in and check in to see how they're going.

Loz Lesson

Ready to find a kick-arse mentor or mastermind to help you grow, develop, and thrive as you achieve your goals? Follow the link to get started.

CLOSING WORDS

You made it! Go you! You're ready.

The greatest gift we have been given is our potential. By setting goals, focusing on our emotional responses to challenges, and taking action towards unlocking our greatest strengths by aligning them with our purpose, we can create an exceptional stack of healthy habits that help us improve the quality of our lives.

We can also… you guessed it… get the f*ck unstuck!

As a coach, it's my job to inspire you to thrive by permitting you to play beyond your wildest dreams. It's my purpose and passion to help you unlock your best self! And to create some kick-arse, healthy habits in the process.

Do you want to know the secret to living your best life? It's pretty simple: just keep on doing Y-O-U!

I am not perfect, but I love that there is absolute beauty in imperfection. Over the years, I've hated myself like you wouldn't believe. Sound familiar? I've been on some pretty epic adventures. I've visited historical places around the world and literally scaled mountains, but none of that made me hate myself any less. Looking back, I realise I didn't appreciate how vital these opportunities to travel and grow were, and I took them for granted. Life-changing, yes – but pivotal? No. Key moments take place in your mind.

Ultimately, my current position in life – where I experience abundance every day – has come from my ability to shift my mindset and establish a critical combination of daily healthy habits that have led to this beautiful place I call now. Know why you're going in a particular direction. Fuel yourself with wholesome goodness. Tune into your inner energies, move your body, practise kindness, and seek mentorship and support. You, too, can realise that the opportunity to feel unique and learn deeply about who you are and where you're travelling exists in every moment.

Your most significant transformation is happening right now. You just have to tap into the moment and realise that it is only right now that you can make it happen.

You have the power (cliché but totally true).

I love that my new-found understanding of how life works has rubbed off on so many people, including my gorgeous husband, Michael. We now share a synergistic lust for life and pay it forward to everyone we meet individually and collectively on our respective journeys. We are living proof that you can achieve anything if you put your mind to it. When you feel aligned on the inside, the outside radiance will naturally flow, and you will look and feel your absolute best. And we have a shit ton of fun doing life together.

I've learnt that the more you praise and celebrate your life, the more there is in life to celebrate. Remember, if you don't celebrate success, it won't mark you! Nothing can dim the light that shines from within. The greatest challenge in life is not discovering who you are… it is being happy with what you find.

Being yourself is more important than being who others expect you to be, so you should stop stressing over others. Always be careful of who you pretend to be because you might forget who you actually are. Stay true to yourself and be proud of who you are, unashamed of how others might see you, because when you stop and look around, this life is pretty damn impressive, and you can be the person you've always wanted to be.

As you arrive at the end of this book, inspired by the idea of healthy new habits, hold onto the fact that you are worthy and enough and unique as you are, but it doesn't mean you need to stay here. It's up to you to live an extraordinary life and not do it half-arsed – it's all about using your complete arse!

WHERE TO NEXT?

My team and I help busy people breathe, hydrate, sleep, eat, and move better to discover unstoppable performance, energy, and confidence for happiness, health, and vitality.

What does that really mean? We can help you move from stuck to unstoppable… and get the f*ck unstuck!

To learn more about Loz Life, Weight Loz, Fab-U Loz, and Boss Loz, and the many programs and tools available to help you on your journey, head to www.lozlife.com, or visit me on social media by searching @lozantonenko, or check out my Loz Life YouTube channel.

In my online shop, I feature a range of valuable tools and resources to help you maintain momentum towards the unstoppable life you deserve.

If you're ready to take your life to the next level, create lifelong vitality, and go deeper to communicate your authentic potential, I invite you to connect with me.

Now spread those wings and soar to great heights… and you'll move from stuck to unstoppable in no time. Peace out for now and, as always, keep it unreal.

IRL (IN REAL LOZ)

By now, you might have realised that I have a lot of weird and wonderful sayings, many of which are scattered throughout this book. In this section, I've compiled the best of the best for you to peruse at your pleasure. Maybe you'll even drop some of them into conversation yourself!

* Nothing tastes as good as healthy feels.

* Shituations.

* Seven-day eventist.

* Infomaniac.

* Helpaholic.

* Me-search over research.

* Simplify to amplify.

* The challenge of action separates the go-getters from the round-to-its.

* Focus is da bomb.

* If you try to fit in, you will never stand out.

* You may not be perfect, but I'll tell you what – you can be awesome.

* Don't worry about the haters who talk behind your back… they're behind you for a reason.

* Let yourself be flawed – it makes for a much more exciting story.

* Sometimes the only difference between kicking arse in life and getting your arse kicked by life is a few positive thoughts followed by a few positive words.

* It's all about having your ducks in a row (as opposed to having ducks that think they're constantly at a rave!).

* Sometimes you have to throw on a crown (or a cape) and remind others who they're dealing with!

* Maybe it's time you stopped 'shoulding' all over yourself.

* The only thing that has to stay where it's planted is a tree.

* I'm not down on dieting, but I am up on nourishing.

* Don't just chase rainbows… eat them!

* Live life to its fullest potential, and fight for your big-arse dreams.

* You are sugar-coating your problems with chocolate, then washing them down with wine.

* No amount of physical strength can match authentic inner prowess (although muscles *are* cute!).

* It's up to you to live an extraordinary life and not do it half-arsed – it's all about using your complete arse!

FURTHER RESOURCE RECOMMENDATIONS

Book List

The Subtle Art of Not Giving a F*ck – Mark Manson
The ONE Thing – Gary Keller and Jay Papasan
The Breakthrough Experience – Dr John Demartini
Unshakeable – Tony Robbins
Positive Intelligence – Shirzad Chamine
Pain Free – Pete Egoscue
Atomic Focus – Patrick McKeown
The 4-Hour Workweek – Tim Ferriss
High Performance Habits – Brendon Burchard
The Secret – Rhonda Byrne
Think Like a Monk – Jay Shetty
The Power of Now – Eckhart Tolle
You Can Heal Your Life – Louise Hay
The Perfect Day Formula – Craig Ballantyne
Super Human – Dave Asprey

Podcast List
The ATP Project
The Demartini Show
Motivation with Brendon Burchard
The Gary Vee Audio Experience
The Tim Ferriss Show
The Human Upgrade with Dave Asprey
She's On The Money
Living 4D with Paul Chek
The Jordan B. Peterson Podcast
The Mindvalley Podcast
The ONE Thing
The Muscle Intelligence Podcast
The Tony Robbins Podcast
Success Resources Podcast
Hintsa High Performance Talks

App List
Muse: meditation & sleep (choosemuse.com/lozlife)
Oura (ouraring.com/taf/651b0b7603)
Asana
Fiverr
BizConnect
Headspace
The Breathing App

Websites List

Calorie Counter Australia – www.caloriecounter.com.au/calorie-calculator

DiSC® personality profiling – www.discprofile.com

Dr John Demartini – www.drdemartini.com

Positive Intelligence – www.positiveintelligence.com

Tony Robbins – www.tonyrobbins.com

Simon Hill (The Proof) – www.theproof.com

Dr Steven Gungry – www.gundrymd.com

Electronic Activity Monitors

Myzone

Polar

Fitbit

Oura

Quality smart watches

Circulation Devices

Theragun

Hyperice

Revitive

Normatec

Other Biohacking Tools

Vielight

Compex

Joovv

Sunlighten saunas

ENAR

ACKNOWLEDGEMENTS

As some of you know, this is the second incarnation of this book, previously called *The Healthy Habit Handbook* when it was first self-published in 2020.

It was a freaking fantastic book, and I received a stack of positive reviews. I was super proud of what I had created. It was a f*cking great first attempt, but I knew I had to do more.

In 2022, I had an aha moment. I have these often, and, ironically, this one was on International Women's Day. I knew I had to rewrite this book, update it, and Lozify it because it wasn't as authentically 'me' as it needed to be.

So, back to my epiphany. I was at an International Women's Day event, listening to author, Lucy Bloom, present. Her book, *Get the Girls Out*, really spoke to me, as did Lucy. She's loud, bright, and full of energy and confidence. What's not to like? She was my kind of woman.

Lucy shared her journey to authorship. Long story short, she accepted an advance from one of the big publishers for her 'business' book. She quickly realised that the daunting task of writing a business book was incredibly overwhelming, and she felt like she couldn't deliver what she had promised. She considered handing back her advance cheque. Serendipitously, after a heartfelt chat with Ariana Huffington's sister, who convinced her to just write "stories about the things you like for the people you love," she found herself spewing out pages and pages of magic with unstoppable gusto. Two years after publishing her memoir under this publishing house, she wanted to do some experimentation with online advertising with the ebook version. Lucy's original publisher kindly handed back all her publishing rights, and she has since published all three of her titles under her own publishing company, Flamingo Publishing. F*ck yeah!

This story made me question my journey and consider how much creative control I wanted over my work. While self-publishing my first book, I worked with one of the big publishing houses' self-publishing arms, and I lost some of myself in the process of trying to fit in. The 'Loz' was watered down. Much of my personality was edited out.

After re-reading it over and over, inherently, my book wasn't authentically Loz. I am brash and crass and like to drop the odd f-bomb. 'Fun' is my second favourite f-word, and my first publication wasn't really a true reflection of what I wanted to say, of my style, or of my vernacular (yep, I like a swear word here and there because they release endorphins in the brain and reduce pain levels – google it). I consider cuss words pattern breakers and attention grabbers, and sometimes my passion needs to be punctuated with a naughty word or two. It's not a sign of a lack of intelligence. It's who I am. I like to suggest that the word 'f*ck' is a simple abbreviation of 'future understanding of conscious knowledge', hence the new title of this book, my updated and overhauled *Healthy Habit Handbook*.

The last few years have been some of the most challenging. I have invested much time and money into creating my unstoppable destiny, working through uncertainty, resilience, pain, and change – beyond my resources' capacity to achieve a more excellent vision than I could have ever imagined.

My book needed to be rewritten because I have been rewritten. My book needed to be more natural, authentic, and vulnerable because I am more real, authentic, and vulnerable.

My vision has changed, and I wanted to share this vision with you all. *Get The F*ck Unstuck!* is a more holistic representation of who I am, where I have been, and where I'm headed. And I'm proud of take two!

But I do need to thank some extraordinary people. And yes, many of them are the same peeps I thanked in my first version of the book. They deserve to be thanked again!

My hunk-of-spunk husband, Michael, has grown into the most incredible partner I couldn't have dreamed up. His thirst for learning has supplied me with an endless well of positivity and encouragement. He's taught me the art of spontaneity and has reminded me that love can evolve as we do. I am so blessed to be able to share in his journey, and I'm grateful that he is sharing in mine. He's funny, brave, and hardworking but knows how to sit in stillness and do absolutely nothing, and I learn from him every single day.

A massive hug to the big guy who has learnt how to reciprocate my embraces with open arms – my life mentor, 'Business' Geoff McDonnell. Our serendipitous meeting at a Tony Robbins event in Sydney in 2018 has led to some equally fortunate opportunities that have allowed me to meet many more fabulous people along the way. Thanks for lighting a dark path with the beam of your radiance, dear friend.

Brian, my beautiful flame – you left this life too soon, yet the candle of your kind and loving heart will be forever etched in the depths of my soul and the legacy I leave when my flesh is but ash. You are the reason for all that is and all that will be.

My family's support is something I do not take for granted. I am genuinely stoked that I have been given such a unique opportunity to grow and express myself alongside a tribe of quirky, sensitive, and non-judgemental relatives, past and present. A big shout-out to my mum, Yvonne, and my two siblings, Amanda and Lochlan. Another big thank you to my father for being one of my great teachers, a silver lining.

Finally, my 'Loz Squad' of A-grade busy bees and coaches who help me take care of business and get all the important stuff done behind the scenes – you know who you are. This passionate squad of creative helpaholics, mentors, and like-minded souls keeps my world turning while I step out of my comfort zone and kick arse daily! Special thanks to Rach, Elle, and Alli for help with this book.

I hope you enjoy reading this book as much as I enjoyed creating it and that it improves your life!

ABOUT THE AUTHOR

LAUREN 'LOZ' ANTONENKO

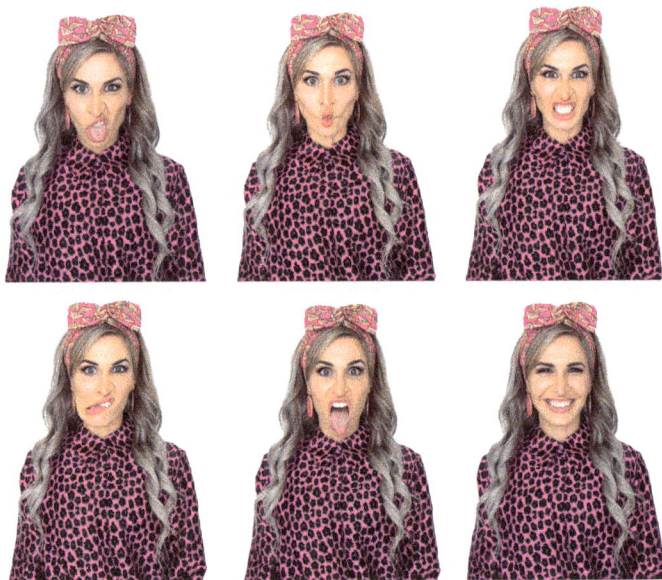

From an early age, Lauren (known as Loz) knew she would live an extraordinary life. She thought she would uncover some magical mystery of the universe or catch a rocket to outer space. Whatever it was, she knew it would be something that would impact the lives of others in a positive, beautiful way.

She grew up in a family of five, the eldest of three kids and the daughter of a nurse mother and military father. As a child, she loved to entertain people, sing and dance on her neighbours' balcony, and put on plays with her outcast group of misfit but kind-natured friends. She always loved to learn and was a tomboy at heart, obsessed with riding BMXs and building high-tech Lego creations. A high achiever from a young age, she played representative basketball, dabbled in musical theatre, and placed highly in track and field sports.

Kids are mean. After changing schools early in her life, Loz was teased for her appearance and for being academically inclined. Luckily, this just fuelled her fire to define herself in other parts of life. She started her first business when she was 15, selling customised name tags for school bags, and this entrepreneurial spirit has stuck with her ever since. Lauren has always had an entrepreneurial fire in her belly.

Upon graduating from high school, Loz was accepted into university on a scholarship and planned to graduate as a software engineer. Halfway through her tertiary studies, however, she grappled with a sexual assault and the sudden onset of chronic illness and was forced to reassess her future career pathway.

Having developed a keen interest in social science and commerce, Loz started a family business with her father in the final year of her undergraduate degree.

Today, she has several business ventures, including that first business (which is still strong) and her self-branded Loz Life world that fosters her highest life values of teaching, learning, and connecting with others.

Despite battling a sea of emotional and physical obstacles, including the suicide of her first husband, a tumour in her brain, and the discovery of a congenital hole in her heart in her early 30s, Loz has overcome a lifetime's worth of challenges. These have led her down a path of self-discovery, self-love, and, ultimately, fulfilment and gratitude. She is a true believer that life happens *for* you, not *to* you.

Having been both overweight and underweight and having struggled with depression and self-sabotage at various stages of her life,

Loz is dedicated to living life to her fullest potential by applying sustainable living practices to her daily routine by way of focusing on optimising what she labels the 'Handbrake Habits': eating, breathing, sleeping, movement, and hydration.

As an award-winning personal trainer, life coach, group fitness and matwork Pilates instructor, weight loss coach, mindfulness specialist, former bikini fitness model, and wellness advocate, Loz is committed to transforming lives by leading her extraordinary life and inspiring others to do the same.

The Healthy Habit Hierarchy is the blueprint she uses to help her clients move from stuck to unstoppable, and this failsafe methodology revolves around the Handbrake Habits.

ENDNOTES

1   Demartini, J 2022, 'A Grateful Mind Opens up a Loving Heart', *Demartini Institute*, viewed 29 September 2023, https://drdemartini.com/blog/grateful-mind-loving-heart.

2   Team Tony, 'The Sustainable Health Diet: A New Approach to Food from Dr. Mark Hyman and Dr. Steven Gundry', *Tony Robbins*, viewed 29 September 2023, https://www.tonyrobbins.com/health-vitality/sustainable-health-diet/.

3   Gundry MD Team 2017, 'The "Gundry Food Strategy"', *Gundry MD,* viewed 29 September 2023, https://gundrymd.com/food-pyramid/.

4   EWG 2016, 'The Pollution in People: Cancer-Causing Chemicals in Americans' Bodies', *EWG*, viewed 30 September 2023, https://www.ewg.org/research/pollution-people.

5   Eske, J 2019, 'How Does Oxidative Stress Affect the Body?', *Medical News Today*, viewed 30 September 2023, https://www.medicalnewstoday.com/articles/324863.php.

6   Carnahan, JC 2018. 'What Is Your Total Toxic Burden? How To Reduce It for Better Health?', *Jill Carnahan,* viewed 30 October 2023, https://www.jillcarnahan.com/2018/07/19/what-is-your-total-toxic-burden-how-to-reduce-it-for-better-health/.

7   Sawani, A, Farhangi, M, Aluganti N, C, Maul, TM, Parsatharathy, S, Smallwood, J & Wei, JL 2018, 'Limiting Dietary Sugar Improves Pediatric Sinonasal Symptoms and Reduces Inflammation', *Journal of Medicinal Food,* vol 21, no 6, pp 527-534, viewed 30 September 2023, 10.1089/jmf.2017.0126.

8   McKeown, P & Macaluso, M 2017, 'Mouth Breathing: Physical, Mental and Emotional Consequences', *Oral Health,* viewed 30 September 2023, https://www.oralhealthgroup.com/features/mouth-breathing- physical-mental-emotional-consequences/.

9   NASPGHAN n.d., 'The Specific Carbohydrate Diet', PDF, Stanford University, viewed 30 September 2023, https://med.stanford.edu/content/dam/sm/gastroenterology/documents/IBD/CarbDiet%20PDF%20final.pdf.

10   Umoh, R 2017, 'Tony Robbins: This Is the No. 1 Skill You Need to Live the Life You Want', *CNBC,* viewed 1 October 2023, https://www.cnbc.com/2017/09/28/tony-robbins-you-need-courage-to-live-the-life-you-want.html.

11   Ajmera, R 2023, '12 Science-Based Benefits of Meditation', *Healthline,* viewed 1 October 2023, https://www.healthline.com/nutrition/12-benefits-of-meditation.

12   Killingsworth, MA & Gilbert, DT 2010, 'A Wandering Mind Is an Unhappy Mind', *Science,* vol 330, p 932, viewed 1 October 2023, https://doi.org/10.1126/science.1192439.

13   Fancy, N 2023, 'The Science of Sleep in Medieval Arabic Medicine: Part 1: Ibn Sīnā's Pneumatic Paradigm', *Consilia Historiae,* vol 163, no 3, pp 662-666, viewed 2 November 2023, https://doi.org/10.1016/j.chest.2022.11.007.

14   Vatansever, F & Hamblin, MR 2012, 'Far Infrared Radiation (FIR): Its Biological Effects and Medical Applications', *Photonics & Lasers in Medicine*, vol, pp 255-266, viewed 1 October 2023, 10.1515/plm-2012-0034.

15   Pall, ML 2018, 'Wi-Fi Is an Important Threat to Human Health', *Environmental Research,* vol 164, pp 405-416, viewed 1 October 2023, doi.org/10.1016/j.envres.2018.01.035.

16   Szabo, S, Yoshida, M, Filakovsky, J & Juhasz, G 2017, '"Stress" Is 80 Years Old: From Hans Selye Original Paper in 1936 to Recent Advances in GI Ulceration', *Current Pharmaceutical Design,* vol 23, no 27, pp 4029-4041, viewed 1 October 2023, 10.2174/1381612823666170622110046.

17   Winzer, EB, Woitek, F & Linke A 2018, 'Physical Activity in the Prevention and Treatment of Coronary Artery Disease', *Journal of the American Heart Association*, vol 7, no 4, viewed 1 October 2023, doi.org/10.1161/JAHA.117.007725.

18   Dempsey, PC, Larsen, RN, Winkler EAH, Owen, N, Kingwell, BA & Dunstan DW 2018, 'Prolonged Uninterrupted Sitting Elevates Postprandial Hyperglycaemia Proportional to Degree of Insulin Resistance', *Diabetes, Obesity and Metabolism*, vol 20, no 6, pp 1526-1530, viewed 1 October 2023, 10.1111/dom.13254.

19   Layne, JE & Nelson, ME 1999, 'The Effects of Progressive Resistance Training on Bone Density: A Review', *Medicine & Science in Sports & Exercise*, vol 3, no 1, pp 25-30, viewed 1 October 2023, 10.1097/00005768-199901000-00006.

20   Cook, L 2019, 'Mental Health in Australia: A Quick Guide', *Parliament of Australia,* viewed 1 October 2023, https://www.aph.gov.au/About%20Parliament/Parliamentary%20 Departments/Parliamentary%20Library/pubs/rp/rp1819/Quick%20Guides/%20Mental-Health.

21   Blumenthal, JA, Smith, PJ & Hoffman, BM 2012, 'Is Exercise a Viable Treatment for Depression?', *ACSM's Health & Fitness Journal,* vol 16, no 4, pp 14-21, viewed 1 October 2023, 10.1249/01.FIT.0000416000.09526.eb.

22   Harvard Health Publishing 2009, 'Counting Every Step You Take', viewed 1 October 2023, https://www.health.harvard.edu/newsletter_article/counting-every-step-you-take.

23   Gardner, B, Lally, P & Wardle, J 2012, 'Making Health Habitual: The Psychology of "Habit-Formation" and General Practice', *The British Journal of General Practice,* vol 62, no 605, pp 664-666, viewed 1 October 2023, 10.3399/bjgp12X659466.

24   CNN 2011, 'Colleagues, Friends React to Steve Jobs' Death', *CNN,* viewed 2 October 2023, https://edition.cnn.com/2011/10/05/us/steve-jobs-reax/index.html.

25   Bolotin, T 2018, 'Fortune 500 Companies Have Mentors, Do You?', *PSA Financial Advisors,* viewed 2 October 2023, www.psafinancial.com/2018/03/most-fortune-500-companies-have-mentor-programs-do-you.

26   Demartini, J 2023, 'Your Perception of Your Success Can Get in the Way of Your Growth', *Demartini Institute,* viewed 2 October 2023, https://drdemartini.com/blog/your-perception-of-success-can-get-in-the-way-of-growth.

27   Demartini, J 2021, 'Dr Demartini on Think and Grow Rich', *Demartini Institute,* viewed 2 October 2023, https://drdemartini.com/blog/dr-demartini-on-think-and-grow-rich.

www.ingramcontent.com/pod-product-compliance
Lightning Source LLC
Chambersburg PA
CBHW052016030426
42335CB00026B/3167